YO IS YOUR BEST BUSINESS WEAPON

THE MINDSMARTS SOLUTION: SCIENCE ON THE RIGHT SIDE OF BUSINESS

KEP KEPNER

Copyright © 2023 by Kep Kepner

All rights reserved. No part of this publication may be reproduced, distributed, or transmitted in any form or by any means without prior written permission.

Kep Kepner -- 1st ed.

ISBN: 978-1-954757-30-1

The Publisher has strived to be as accurate and complete as possible in the creation of this book.

This book is not intended for use as a legal, business, accounting, or financial advice source. All readers are advised to seek the services of competent professionals in legal, business, accounting, and finance fields.

Like anything else in life, there are no guarantees of income or results in practical advice books. Readers are cautioned to rely on their judgment about their individual circumstances to act accordingly.

While all attempts have been made to verify information provided in this publication, the Publisher assumes no responsibility for errors, omissions, or contrary interpretation of the subject matter herein. Any perceived slights of specific persons, peoples, or organizations are unintentional.

FOREWORD

Three years ago, Kep Kepner, CPA, came to the Center for BrainHealth at the University of Texas at Dallas (UTD) to discover whether our High-Performance Brain Training had direct applications to benefit his business insights as well as to support his clients as small business owners better. As a CPA, he has coached many small business owners and witnessed how they become stuck or slow to adapt to help their businesses change and thrive with the times. He was looking for solutions. We were looking for someone who could develop direct applications of brain strategies to CPAs. The team effort is bringing about a trifecta win – for BrainHealth, Kep, and now for YOU.

Kep experienced measurable gains after completing the training and actively implementing the mental strategy toolkit. Not only did he personally improve as measured by his BrainHealth Index, but he also reported that his revenues, profits, and bottom-line ROI increased significantly, with new possibility thinking and habits toward key decisions and tasks. The additive value of his High-Performance Brain Training was that he could do more with less effort by re-calibrating his mental energy, freeing time to create MindSmarts.com. What is impressive about Kep is that he leads, motivates, and inspires others.

Since its formation in 1999, UTD Center for BrainHealth has become the world's leading neuroscience institution focused on understanding how the brain works and can be strengthened at any age, thanks to the brain's immense modifiability (neuroplasticity). Our goal is to bring Brain Health measurement and solutions to the world. The science of brain health has more than 600 clinical studies to provide a solid foundation for our work. Similar to the introduction of heart health awareness 20 years ago, awareness of brain health is growing throughout the world today. The problem is individuals do not know where to turn for brain health solutions. The BrainHealth Team is working tirelessly to change the conversation and increase accessibility to protocols that build better brain health.

Center for BrainHealth is leading a landmark study that seeks to enroll, annually monitor, coach, and train 120,000 healthy adults (10 to 100 years) to see how successfully brain health can be promoted, maintained, and improved year to year. One of the key contributions of the BrainHealth Project is an evidenced-based BrainHealth Index, a multi-dimensional metric comprising three key factors of **clarity, connectedness to people, and purpose and emotional balance** that support one's ability to thrive in their context. The Index is being linked to neural changes that correspond to improved brain performance, such as that achieved by High-Performance Brain Training. We are beginning to measure the upward potential of the human mind to move beyond simply identifying deficits, disease-onset and progression, and losses of brain capacity.

Like most institutions, our early studies centered on finding solutions for medically related brain issues, such as brain injury, dementia, mental health, and more. We expanded our discovery to address whether healthy people could benefit. The answer is a resounding YES. The science of brain health now makes clear that when a brain functions well, people perform well. Brain health as studied by the Center for BrainHealth, focuses on cognitive, emotional, and social resources. Improvement in brain health leads to greater resilience, fortitude, and clarity, human qualities that improve an individual's ability to flourish in their personal and professional life.

As the world continues to change at a dizzying pace, these human qualities of resilience, fortitude, and clarity guide people to adapt to the pace of change and improve their brain resources simultaneously. According to Kep, business owners already have a high level of fortitude and resilience but still, become stuck in their businesses. We believe our brain performance protocols can enhance their business decision-making and strategic actions.

In this book, Kep applies High-Performance Brain Training as a significant part of the advisory services he offers through KepnerCPA, making this approach unique in the business community. The business problems he has selected to discuss are common business issues that all businesses face from time to time. His advisory practice centers on giving business owners proven advice to meet their objectives. Armed with the knowledge of High-Performance Brain Training, business owners will better understand the problems they are facing and the alternative decisions they may make for the betterment of their business.

Kep speaks from personal experience, not just textbook answers. We are both curious to see how far you can take our brain strategies and the applications to stretch your mind and fuel greater success. To what degree will you take the personal challenge to see if you can better use your greatest assets – your agile and innovative brain skills - to thrive as your business grows?

I look forward to hearing personal stories about how you benefit from our brain tools and Kep's counsel!

Yours,

Sandra Bond Chapman, Ph.D.
Founder and Chief Director, Center for BrainHealth

Dee Wyly, Distinguished University Professor
The University of Texas at Dallas

CONTENTS

Introduction: Why Is a CPA Talking About Brain Health? ix

Chapter 1	The Trapped Business Owner 1	
Chapter 2	Brain Science and Performance: Strategic Attention 17	
Chapter 3	Brain Science and Performance: Integrated Reasoning 29	
Chapter 4	Brain Science and Performance: Innovation 37	
Chapter 5	Roadmap 47	
Chapter 6	Pricing Your Product 59	
Chapter 7	Cash Flow 65	
Chapter 8	Marketing 101 79	
Chapter 9	Financing Your Business 91	
Chapter 10	What Keeps You up at Night? 105	
Chapter 11	Using High Brain Performance on Personal Matters 113	
Appendix A	The Ideal Client Scene for Kepner CPA 123	
Appendix B	41 Marketing Strategies 127	

About Kep Kepner, CPA, CEPA 129
What Kep's Clients are Saying 131

INTRODUCTION

WHY IS A CPA TALKING ABOUT BRAIN HEALTH?

Everything we do is preceded by a thought, either a conscious thought or an unconscious reaction. As a CPA, I became fascinated with the brain 30 years ago as I saw my business clients doing the same things repeatedly and expecting different results. I believe this is the definition of "insanity."

As CPAs, we have a unique role with our clients. Many of them stay with us for years, so we can see their decision-making and measure their results in financial terms. Because we are considered trusted advisors to our clients, we are privy to financial information and family and personal matters.

In addition, because we have a degree of separation from our clients, we can see things in their lives that they cannot see. This is true of most professionals with an objective view of their clients. In our case, however, we can see their decision process and learn the results of those decisions through a financial window. I am often amazed at the thought processes. If people could only approach their problems differently, they would get better results.

The result for many is the trap of short-term thinking. This type of thinking and decision-making traps people in deciding for the short term at the sacrifice of the strategic life needed in this rapidly changing world. I see this as being **"trapped by the familiar."** It can be explained as **"life getting in the way of our plans."**

I looked for solutions because many of our clients wanted to decide for themselves even though they had a trusted advisor on their side. Several of them still go alone, without our help. One of my friends, a financial planner, said, "Kep, sometimes they just stop listening to me!" when advising clients on saving and investment strategies that would help them. I concluded that if I could help our clients, mainly small business owners, make better decisions on their own, that would be my legacy contribution to the world.

SO WHAT IS BRAIN HEALTH?

Brain Health is essential for everyone. The studies from the Center for BrainHealth of the University of Texas at Dallas give us important scientific knowledge through 600 clinical studies from over 100 neuroscientists that tell us about the brain:

- We start to lose our cognitive capital beginning in our twenties. Think about the plaque that builds up in our arteries from burgers and fries but only shows up when we have to go to the cardiologist in our 60s. We don't notice it until we get older.
- We can regain any lost cognitive capital that we have lost. Once we know it is lost, we can recover it simply by thinking differently about the things that are important to us. We

bring to the table these High-Performance tools to foster self-improvement.
- Modern medicine has allowed us to measure our cognitive resources and brain changes through MRIs and other tests. The Center for BrainHealth can measure the growth in the brain and the increased blood flow that results during and after High-Performance Brain Training. You can see these changes yourself by simply observing your own performance.
- Our chronological age far surpasses our brain power, which may leave some of us unable to care properly for ourselves. Many of us will live to age 100 or older, but our loss of cognitive resources catches up to us in our 60s.
- Our brains are constantly changing. The scientific term is "brain plasticity." The brain changes for the better if used properly and for the worse if not.
- We can be in control of our brains. The choices we make in how we use our brains give us control; all we need are the simple tools to follow.

My laboratory for 30 years has included thousands of small businesses. Most of them start with a dream. Perhaps just to be on their own. Maybe to build a global empire. I know this; a spirited entrepreneur committed to their idea can change the world. But along the way, many get lost. As a result of the demands on them, they become trapped by the same business that was their dream; they begin to think day-to-day, not long-term.

It is as if they have forgotten how to think strategically, faced with the reality of the financial and time commitment to make it happen. This commitment is needed for both the global business and the local business. Both require long-term strategic thinking.

We all make short-term decisions at the expense of long-term strategies. So why is the business owner or entrepreneur unique? Because they were willing to be creative and strategic and to take the risks of starting their enterprise. They are the heart of American business. That is why they represent a unique group. If they become trapped, it isn't easy to recapture those traits that allowed them to become entrepreneurs in the first place.

The program I have developed after partnering with the Center for BrainHealth and its founder, Sandra Bond Chapman, author of "Make Your Brain Smarter," is called MindSmarts. This series of training workshops focuses on "High-Performance Brain Training" and business content to help business owners reclaim their power, refine their focus, and get back to the roots of their passion for entrepreneurship. Join me as we explore your most powerful business weapon - **your brain.**

- Kep Kepner

CHAPTER 1

THE TRAPPED BUSINESS OWNER

As a CPA and a small business owner, I am uniquely positioned to understand and recognize a "Trapped Business Owner." I have been one myself from time to time. As a CPA, I am a trusted advisor for many small business owners. I can see at a close and personal level, from a personal relationship and from their financial information, when they are stuck or trapped. They often don't recognize it, even though they feel the results.

This has been my laboratory for my entire business career; coupled with the coaching of over 1,000 business owners, I have seen and understand a lot about these unique creatures, the business owners. As an outside advisor, I have always been able to spot what is wrong in a business; usually, it starts with the owner. The owner is ingrained in their business. Their personality and decision-making are reflected in how they live their lives and how their business performs.

As such, they often can't see the changes that will benefit their company. In many cases, this is because "change" means "more work" for them. They are already too busy. Much is made about meeting the owner where they are. This typically relates to their age. The Baby Boomers (1946-1964) invented the 60-hour work week; they are tired. The GenXers (1965-1980) want work/life balance. The Millennials (1981-2000) earn to spend; they will learn their lessons later in life when they don't have anything. Gen Z (2000-2025) is the technology wizards; their short attention spans and lack of focus will hinder them.

Regardless of their generation, all business owners can become trapped. The challenge for most will be to recognize it. Once recognized, they have to strategize. Once strategizing, they have to implement change. Once they implement change, they must measure and monitor it in the ever-changing world. It is a difficult task for anyone. Until someone experiences some pain or aspires to a greater existence, they may live trapped and not recognize it. It is what it is!

What are the signs of someone who is trapped? They are varied and different. We have seen evidence of an employee coming home from work frazzled, worn out, and unfulfilled. Same problem; different day. That is worse for the business owner. Employees can moan and complain about their boss, employer, and company decisions. These are often things that the employee can't control. But what about the business owner? The owner can't complain without pointing the finger at themselves. So they often go down that river in Egypt, de Nile.

When they are worn out, unfilled, and bored, it is difficult to drum up the energy necessary to make changes. They may not know why (they really do if they are honest with themselves), but they feel this lack of energy, the lack of fulfillment, and the competing demands of work and family.

Remember, no matter how they enter the business world, business owners are different from other people in business. They usually start their business with a dream. They also have the ability to take risks. Over time as they make compromise after compromise, the dream fades. Over time other demands are made on them, and they forget what brought them to that business in the first place. **They begin living off of it, not feeding it. It becomes a lifestyle business, not an investment of value.**

Let's go back to when they started. Sometimes they just thought they could perform better than those they worked for. "I am better than my boss." Let's start with the assumption that they are better than their boss. That only describes what the work is, the product, and the service. It doesn't mean that someone is a business owner; they are just a worker.

A lone wolf contract worker can earn a lot of money; however, that is not running a business. If you are an IT professional working on a company's computer structure, the first thing you may run into is the need to provide broader services, such as website design. If you don't have that skill (maybe more of a marketing skill than related to technology), a competitor does. And by the way, that competitor has an IT person to compete for the business you are doing. You could become stuck and held hostage by your largest (only) customer.

Now instead, say you take on a few more clients. You don't feel like you are being held hostage anymore. Feeling good, you hire someone to help. They take a big load off of you, and you relax. That is until you see that they can do as well as you, and they may take some of that business away from you. Or they take a load off of you, but you must spend more time training and managing this worker. You become stuck because you are not as connected to your customers, and you have to correct or explain your worker's work. Now you are being held hostage by your employee.

Perhaps you had the worker on contract, but he had tax problems and called the Department of Labor, the Unemployment Commission, or the IRS and complained that he thought you were taking money for taxes out of his pay. Now you have more burdens placed on you, and you are stuck again. You are pissed and have to replace the worker but pay taxes on who you hire. Now you are held hostage by the government.

You get past that since you only have one employee, but you are back to square one with more costs. You find a great solution; unfortunately, the new hero costs more than you can afford, so you pop over to your friendly banker to get some money, but this is the first time you have done that. They are nice, but they can't loan you any money because, trying to lower your tax bill, you wrote off all kinds of expenses, and the bank can't see how you can afford to pay them back. Somehow, you convince them to loan you some cash. Now you are held hostage by the bank.

The gist of this learning experience of becoming a business owner is that your plate is full with each step (either forward or backward). It is somewhat like the movie, *The Godfather*. "Just when I thought I was out, they pull me back in!" So goes your life with a business that continues to require all of what you have to give. How do you know if you are making progress or just treading water? As a practical matter, ask yourself:

1. Do I have enough take-home pay for my personal life?
2. Do I have funds to invest back in my business?

3. Am I current on all business obligations (bank loans, credit cards, regular payables)?
4. Am I current on all personal obligations (mortgage, car payments, credit cards, etc.)?
5. Have I developed a savings or investment program for kids, college, or retirement?

If not, take heart. You may recoup it when you are ready to sell and retire. Many owners find that their business is not worth what they thought it would be, and they can't really retire. They have spent so much time on their business that they have yet to invest outside of their business and rely on it to support their lifestyle.

What they miss is that despite being trapped or stuck in their business, there are opportunities to break out of that spiral. But who can they turn to?

Their spouse: If the spouse is active in the business, they are also trapped.

Their family: The business owner doesn't want to admit to their family that they are trapped.

Their employees: The business owner thinks, "They work for me, don't they?"

Their banker: If the business owner seems distressed, the banker might lose confidence and not renew the loans.

Their CPA: The business owner thinks, "Don't they just do my books and tax return?"

Their lawyer: The business owner thinks, "Will they really know what to do?"

Their friends at the club (church, neighborhood, you name it): The business owner doesn't want to look bad, so they carry that burden and put on a brave smiling face.

The owner has to turn back to the one person they trust or want to trust. Themselves. To make the best decisions, the business owner can benefit from implementing the High-Performance Brain Training described at MindSmarts.com. That may be enough. If not, they need someone to give them objectivity. With High-Performance thinking and the benefit of an objective point of view, they can recapture what they may have lost.

The very personality traits that caused them to choose to go into the business are the traits that keep them trapped. Their dependence only on themselves results in having no one to talk to and no one to trust to give them objective advice. Their brave face to take the risk of a business causes them to depend on themselves without the skills to adapt as things change. The joy of achievement is replaced with doubt when they learn the business is not worth as much as they desire.

To make things easier, they tell everyone they make decisions by their "gut." They don't need to look at financials; they don't need to measure activities; they concentrate on the customers. They don't waste time on what trends are happening; the current needs trump being strategic.

If that is how you operate, you aren't held hostage by anyone except yourself and your beliefs. And you find you *have* to go to work, not that you *want* to go to work. No wonder others are waiting for you to act. Not only are you stuck, but others become stuck as well. Don't get me wrong. Owning a business is exciting, challenging, fun, and rewarding, just not consistently. The business owner knows what they know, but there is a lot of business activity that they need help understanding. If I own a business and am making $350K per year, my business life, my family life, and my individuality may be great. The world is moving fast and can destroy a business in just a few years. Consider a taxi driver or a taxi company in NYC. Two years and gone.

Are you brave enough to take a simple test as to whether you are trapped or stuck in your business? I challenge you to do so. The good news is that by investing back into what got you here, **YOU**, you can begin to make progress and build your business and life, so you are in control again. Using the protocols for High-Performance Brain Training, you can regain that control and begin to make long-term and strategic decisions. If you find a trusted advisor, you can use these protocols to act on what you discover about your business and life.

Are you Stuck (Or Trapped)?
On a scale of 1-10, answer "1" if you are trapped; "10" if you are in control.

Are you getting the same results from your business as always, no matter what you do? (Comment: Answer high if you are getting the same results and it is alright, i.e., the money is okay, and you are still energized. Answer low if the results aren't enough.)

1	2	3	4	5	6	7	8	9	10
Everything stays the same, or results are not enough				Get different results				Get different results that are great!	

Is this complex world moving too fast with business issues you are unprepared for? (Comment: There may be new technology and competitors, and you must make investments to prepare for these. Answer high if you are on top of these challenges; no sweat.)

1	2	3	4	5	6	7	8	9	10
I can't keep up Too tired Cost is too much				I'll find a way Tired, little energy Eventually I will do it				Love challenges Bring it on I will do it!	

Do you feel like you are treading water? (Comment: Do you feel like nothing changes no matter your business decisions? Answer low if you are treading water and every decision you make seems to create more work for you and high if you are always making progress.)

1	2	3	4	5	6	7	8	9	10
I am sinking				I'll find a way				Walking on water	

Do you go home at night worn out and unfulfilled? (Comment: You have important things to do and can't get to them. You are too busy and never have time for yourself. Being hopeful, you hope it will be temporary. Answer low if you are worn out, high if you are energized.)

1	2	3	4	5	6	7	8	9	10
I am sinking				Sometimes it is ok					I am energized

Do you always seem to need cash for your business or family? (Comment: There doesn't seem to be enough money for your business or family commitments, and you have been unable to plan for those needs. You see prices going up, and your costs are increasing, but you can't seem to raise your prices. Answer low if this is you.)

1	2	3	4	5	6	7	8	9	10
Never enough				Up and down					I have enough

Has the bank turned you down, or do you have creditors hounding you for any reason? (Comment: Sometimes bank requirements are so daunting that it feels like they are turning you down; it will take a lot of work to get the financing you need. Answer low if this is your life.)

1	2	3	4	5	6	7	8	9	10
They are bloodsuckers				They are there when needed					I have what I need

Do your measurements seem contradictory to your gut feel? (Comment: Do you make a trade-off by looking at financial statements or metrics, wondering what they mean or what actions to take, mainly when there is insufficient money? Answer low if contradictory and high if they align with your gut.)

1	2	3	4	5	6	7	8	9	10
I don't understand, so I use my gut				I measure what I need to			My gut feel is validated by my metrics		

Do you feel captive by third parties that are important to your business? (Comment: Do you have to drop everything or change your priorities because of demands from your largest customers, your vendors, your employees, the IRS, or others? Answer low if you are captive to anyone.)

1	2	3	4	5	6	7	8	9	10
Yes, customers, employees, Uncle Sam				I can work through it				No one holds me hostage	

Do you have the energy and time to develop a roadmap to improve your business? (Comment: According to Yogi Berra, "If you don't know where you are going, you will end up somewhere else." Putting together a plan is hard work. Your goals are the destination; your roadmap is the "how." Answer low if you don't have a roadmap or don't know how to be strategic.)

1	2	3	4	5	6	7	8	9	10
No, I don't know how				I can learn				I am following my roadmap	

Is your new business pipeline empty, so you feel like you are just starting again and again? (Comment: Different day, same problems. Knowing your pipeline is draining, particularly when you have mouths to feed. Answer low if you constantly have to start over.)

1	2	3	4	5	6	7	8	9	10
I have to start over				Business comes and goes				Operating according to my plan	

Is your new business pipeline too full when you are already overloaded with work? (Comment: How can you respond to new business when you already have money, people, backlog, supply chain, or vendor problems? It might be a good problem unless it falls back on you. Answer low if you are tired.)

1	2	3	4	5	6	7	8	9	10
Too Busy; too tired				I will get a break soon				I have plans on how to overcome	

Are you having a problem hiring the right people? (Comment: It is not just hiring people but finding the good ones. When you find good people, are you fearful that they may leave, putting a burden back on you because no one works as hard as you? Answer low if you have "people problems" and can't seem to resolve them.)

1	2	3	4	5	6	7	8	9	10
More people; more problems				Hope I choose a good one				I always find good people	

Does your to-do list look the same every morning? (Comments: You have too many demands from too many people, and you have important tasks that never seem to be completed. "We have always done it that way. The last time I tried it, it didn't work. Too many choices; how can I choose?" These may just be excuses. You probably know you are too busy if the list looks the same and you don't know how to prioritize. Answer low if your to-do list looks the same as yesterday.)

1	2	3	4	5	6	7	8	9	10
The same; important things don't get done				Get things done, not the best			I get the important things done as needed		

Are other people stuck because you can't get things done? (Comments: Sometimes, people cannot get things done that are important to you because you are the bottleneck. Sometimes people cannot make progress on things that are important to them because you are the bottleneck. If so, people may think less of you because they can't count on you. Answer low if you are slowing others down.)

1	2	3	4	5	6	7	8	9	10
It's my company I'm a bottleneck				People need to get things done They don't have to wait for me			We operate so everyone is respected and gets things done as needed		

Do you have anyone that you can trust to help you? (Comments: It isn't enough to have someone to trust; they must have your best interests in mind, whether an employee, a coach, a family member, a business group, or someone else. Answer high if you have someone to trust or if you can fully trust yourself.)

1	2	3	4	5	6	7	8	9	10
I don't want them to know my weaknesses and problems I have no one to trust				I don't have anyone to count on Everyone seems to want money What's in it for them?			I trust myself fully or have proven advisors who give me objectivity		

Are you afraid to tell people your "secret sauce" even though you can't get around to implementing it? (Comments: If you have great ideas about your business but cannot implement them, it may be due to a promise you made to yourself when you started the business. It could also mean your business is not different from any other in your industry. Answer low if your secret sauce is so secret it won't see the light of day.)

1	2	3	4	5	6	7	8	9	10
Don't have a secret sauce Don't want someone else to steal it				I am working on it but I haven't announced it yet; hopefully, soon			I can protect my secret sauce so I promote it because everyone is too busy to steal it		

Are you long-term and strategic in your business decisions? (Comment: Being strategic does not always result in the gains a business expects; do you want to take such a risk? Think about whether you are building an enterprise or just living off your business. Answer low if you are living off your business.)

1	2	3	4	5	6	7	8	9	10
I have to worry about Friday payroll. I don't have time to think or be strategic				I'm stuck in the short term. I have to survive first and need help. I'm lost			I make long and short-term decisions that keep me on top of my business.		

Are you going to work because you want to or because you have to? (Comment: Being bored, lonely, distracted, tired, or upset with yourself is an emotional response that puts you in a victim mindset and suggests you cannot find good solutions. The same is said if you think you can solve your problems by being more disciplined. Answer low if you have to go to work.)

1	2	3	4	5	6	7	8	9	10
Don't want to; must				Sometimes want; always must			Energized; always want		

Is your family suffering because of your work demands? (Comment: You know the answer to this. You and your spouse disagree on your choice of work. You haven't saved for retirement, your kid's college, or your life, and you feel like you have failed. Answer low if suffering.)

1	2	3	4	5	6	7	8	9	10
They suffer from my business demands				Sometimes I am not there			I have a healthy family life balance		

Do you not know what your business is worth, or do you know the worth, and that's not enough? (Comment: Too often, business owners wait until they are going to retire to find out that their business, the one that they put their heart and soul into, is not worth enough to retire on. Answer low if you don't know the worth or know it isn't worth much.)

1	2	3	4	5	6	7	8	9	10
No clue really				General business stats			Valuation within a year		

Have you lost focus on your business? (Comment: Lack of focus has killed far more businesses than lack of capital. Answer low if you are unfocused.)

1	2	3	4	5	6	7	8	9	10
No clue really				General business stats			Valuation within a year		
Always distracted									

As a practical matter, you may not recognize if you are trapped. Sometimes being trapped is good. If you make enough money to live and save for the future, you can be fulfilled while trapped. The real measurement often comes when you realize your business has little value outside of you, so it simply provides a living and cannot be sold for an amount needed to retire. Doesn't it make sense to do something about it now? See where you stand.

Score	Reasoning
21-50	You are trapped; how do you get out of your bed in the morning?
51- 130	There is hope, hope that you will come to your senses.
131-170	With some new tools and a roadmap, you can do great.
171-190	You are on track to do good things.
190-210	You are invigorated and wise in following your plan.

CHAPTER

2

BRAIN SCIENCE AND PERFORMANCE: STRATEGIC ATTENTION

Strategic attention is all about endurance, the equivalent of endurance in physical training. It's priming your brain for optimal performance. An athlete doesn't just go out and run the race. They do all kinds of warm-ups. They have a method where they visualize running the race, observe their competitors, and look at the conditions around their activity. In doing so, they prime themselves for optimal performance before they begin. That's precisely what strategic attention entails. There are three protocols you're going to learn, the first one being the "brainpower of two."

THE BRAINPOWER OF TWO

Pause for a minute and pull out your to-do list for the day. Maybe your list is on a yellow pad. Perhaps it's on the computer. Maybe it's in your brain and not on paper anymore. But take a look at that to-do list. Ask yourself and be honest, "Are there items that have been on there for weeks?" I know that my to-do list encounters this problem from time to time. Sometimes I go home at the end of the day, and I don't feel like I accomplished much of anything; I don't feel fulfilled. After all, there will be a new batch of emails tomorrow after I've disposed of the current ones. And the phone will still ring tomorrow. What about that stack of papers on your desk? What about those jobs that you still need to get to? What about the tools in your toolbox that need to be cleaned or prepared for the next day?

So we all have these to-do lists, but we make big mistakes when dealing with them. Here's the way to approach your to-do list using the brainpower of two. "When you're hunting elephants, don't get distracted by chasing rabbits." You might wonder what elephants and rabbits have to do with the topic at hand. Well, this didn't come from some nerdy accountant in my office or the scientific labs at the Center for BrainHealth. This quote came from Boone Pickens. Who was Boone Pickens? Boone Pickens was a billionaire. He was a corporate raider. He owned various major companies and said, "When you're hunting elephants, don't get distracted by chasing rabbits."

There's a corollary to this. If you're chasing rabbits, you're not going to catch any of them because they will come back tomorrow. So think about this when you're tackling important, big things. Don't let yourself get distracted. The brainpower of two says, "Identify two high-priority items to get done every day." The elephants are the major tasks you tackle when your brain is at its best. For many, it is the first thing in the morning instead of later in the day. These are priorities that require higher-order thinking. Higher-order thinking includes complex problem-solving, innovative thinking, mental flexibility, judgment, analysis, measurement, decision-making, social adeptness, and stress regulation. Does answering an email require higher-order thinking? No. In my case, does doing a tax return like the thousands I have done throughout my career require higher-order thinking? No, because I know how to do it.

The key is to prioritize two difficult things that require you to think deeply and broadly. Each of these needs to be accomplished within 45 minutes. You might think, "Why 45 minutes? I have an elephant that I've got to slay. It will take me all day." The reason for 45 minutes is that it is about the length of time that your brain can concentrate on a particular important matter at its best. When you need a break after 45 minutes in a workshop or meeting, your brain gets tired, and you stop using your strong resources.

The other essential element to your top priorities is that they must move your needle forward professionally or personally. Let's say, in my world, I have a major tax return to review after one of my staff completes it. That may be an important task. It may have to be done by a deadline because a client is leaving town or needs to make business decisions by knowing the answers. That might be something that moves the needle forward for somebody who's learning how to do tax returns. But for me, that's probably not moving my needle forward. What's moving my needle forward most recently has been working on applying brain training to help my clients grow. So when I spend time doing work that I'm expected to know how to do and mundane work, like emails and communications, those are not moving my needle forward. Sure, they may be necessary. After all, we've got to keep doing good work and making our clients happy.

But we have to focus on the broader picture as well. The brainpower of two tells you to choose two elephants each day, which will be uniquely different for each of us. Ensure that they require higher-order thinking, you can accomplish them in 45 minutes, and they are priorities that move your needle forward.

Think about it for a minute. If you spend all day answering emails, what has that really done for you? You are not using your brain to its fullest capacity. Think about it when you go home at night. If you have accomplished something significant that moved you forward personally, learned something new, applied something new, or made progress on something important to you, those are the nights you fall asleep feeling good. If you feel drained and your brain is exhausted, it's because you did mundane work that didn't require you to use your full capabilities. You were worn out by the mediocre tasks distracting you from the big picture, or the elephant, as the case may be.

PRACTICING WITH THE BRAINPOWER OF TWO

It's time to put what you've learned about the brainpower of two into practice. I also want you to think about the activities in your frontal lobe because that's where your growth occurs. It's the executive network that manages your life, your higher-level thinking, and the way you operate.

The two "elephants" on your to-do list require strategy, analysis, and heavy-duty thinking, all of which occur in the frontal lobe. These are the tasks that will move your needle forward. On the business front, the first elephant in this example is an annual review for an employee. Now think about that. That has to be strategic. You think deeply about what the employee has done, how their performance has affected other people in the company, whether they have reached goals for themselves, and what you can do to help them achieve more to the benefit of themselves and the company. So, doing an annual review for somebody takes a lot of planning, strategy, and analysis. Those are the kinds of things your brain likes. And if you do that review and go home at night, you'll feel like you accomplished something. Even if it's a negative review, you're going to feel like you got that major thing off your desk (or your back) and have a plan for what to do and follow up.

Now, what about your Uncle Jack's birthday party? You still have that to plan. Where's it going to be? Who's going to be invited? Does it require travel plans? Does it need various kinds of presents, food, or entertainment? Again, you have to be strategic about this task. How long do you have before Uncle Jack's birthday? You'll probably take him out for a burger if it's tomorrow. But suppose it's a month from now. In that case, you're going to engage in some deep planning activities that are important to move your needle forward in terms of your relationship with your family, your role in the family, and your relationship with Uncle Jack.

Both of these examples are elephants that require using your brain deeply to cover all the bases. Of course, those rabbits will be hopping around and distracting you. You could probably check emails all day long. I've learned how to assign some of my emails to other people. Staff meetings can be rabbits, too, unless you are responsible for planning the meeting or covering a critical or sensitive topic. So a particular activity could be a rabbit today that turns into an elephant later.

Activities like scheduling doctor's appointments, having lunch with a friend to talk about the Dallas Cowboys, or picking up the kids from school don't require heavy-duty brain work. But what if these rabbits are distracting you? The fact is, you can only pay attention to one thing at a time. For example, pretend I gave you an article to read about the sleep patterns of dolphins and whales while simultaneously I read an article out loud about the effects of marijuana use. It would be challenging to answer if I asked you questions about the content of both articles when we were done reading. How many participants were in the marijuana study? Why do dolphins and whales sleep differently than humans? Most likely, you will be scratching your head, especially since most people in this situation will zone out on the less interesting topic of the two.

Can you relate this scenario to things going on in your office right now? You're concentrating on something significant to you, a client, or a staff member. And somebody interrupts you to talk about baseball scores. That may be more interesting right now. So you might be drawn away from the more important task at hand.

You also have to know where you're going when talking about elephants. For some, that may come in the form of goals. I have people in my firm studying for the CPA exam, which will undoubtedly move their needles forward personally and professionally. I prefer to use the term "roadmap" instead of "goals." Yogi Berra, the New York Yankee Hall of Fame Manager, once said, "If you don't know where you're going, you're going to end up somewhere else." It works the same way with your thinking. To set the proper foundation for your elephants, you need to know where you're going.

THE BRAINPOWER OF ONE

I love when I receive a resume from someone wanting to work at my CPA firm or MindSmarts, and they open with, "I'm very good at multitasking." I know they're not, and it's very easy to prove.

Remember the last example about trying to comprehend two separate articles about marijuana use and marine life? Our brains aren't wired for multitasking.

What does multitasking really mean? Multitasking is doing two or more tasks simultaneously and pursuing separate goals at the same time. Let's take some paperwork and an interrupter at my door as an example. The goal of my paperwork is to complete a project, while the goal of the person interrupting me is to have me engage in whatever they want to talk about.

Multitasking is NOT being responsible for multiple tasks or projects or using different modalities to accomplish the same goal. I have a lot of things that I'm responsible for during the day as I run my company. But being responsible for multiple tasks or projects is not multitasking. Having many components to one project is not multitasking.

For example, to get MindSmarts up and running, I had to develop a logo and trademark it. I had to make sure that I could obtain www.mindsmarts.com. I had to develop a website. I had to create all the materials available on the website and learn how to record the information. I had to coordinate with the Center for BrainHealth. Regarding technical matters, I had to be prepared for people who wanted to use the website in a way I had not thought of. And then I had to make the whole thing operational. Even though all of this work related to one project, that wasn't multitasking. There were many different components or elephants to the same project over several months. The goal was the same.

What are the effects of multitasking? Chronic multitasking is toxic to your brain. Your brain is not wired for it. It makes you a sucker for irrelevancy. If I'm in my office working on something important, and my colleague pops in to talk about the game on Sunday, it's hard to get back on track. My thinking becomes shallower, and I am more error-prone because it leads to a decline in fluid intelligence. We all have fixed intelligence, which is our knowledge base, for example, tax law or engineering. Fluid intelligence is applying our fixed knowledge to situations in today's world that affect us. If fluid intelligence declines, it leads to significant brain atrophy and chronic stress.

The brainpower of one means limiting multitasking and sequencing tasks one at a time versus trying to do multiple tasks at once. Another part is filtering out unnecessary things, blocking out unimportant information, and eliminating distractions. Turn off your cell phone when you're in your office working on something. Close the door. If you're working from home, go to a different room or outside. Do something to limit the interruptions that will hinder your ability to resolve major issues.

Let's look at this by the numbers. Some of the statistics are amazing to me. One to three minutes is the average time most people can work without interruption or switching tasks. It's hard to believe any of us ever get anything done! I can't do anything in three minutes other than answer a simple email. 20 to 25 minutes is the average time to resume focus after interruption. And 38% of the time, people don't even go back to what they were working on before they were interrupted. It's easy to see why that relates to a 40% decrease in productivity due to distractions and multitasking.

You have a lot of control over your life. Shut the door. Turn off the phone. Identify an elephant you are going to work on. Work on that elephant for 45 minutes; get it done so you can feel good about the day. Then open your door or answer all those emails that flood your inbox, which don't move your needle forward personally or professionally. I know my wife is frequently interrupted by her phone. She's in sales, and her cell phone is the conduit to her clients. So in her case, I'm sure she looks at her phone 150 times a day. Her elephants come from holding her calls and completing major client projects. But I have it easier because I have greater control over my environment. And I'm much more productive. I use the power of one to limit multitasking, and I create an environment in my office space where I can accomplish something without interruption.

THE BRAINPOWER OF NONE

When do you most often experience "aha" moments? When does the light bulb turn on? For me, it's usually in the morning when I'm relaxed and refreshed. Some people have "aha" moments in the shower, when they exercise, when they interact with nature, or after meditation. There's no "right" answer to when it happens to you. But boy, when you identify one of those "aha" moments, it feels incredible because now you've uncovered something you have been searching for. This usually doesn't happen during periods of high stress.

What happens when you're stressed? You have an inundation of cortisol, the hormone that creates more stress and leads to chronic stress. You also experience reduced amounts of dopamine; the "feel good" chemical in your brain. Think back on a time when you accomplished something significant. Remember how good you felt? That was a shot of dopamine.

The brainpower of none is a way of recharging your cognitive energy throughout the day and exploiting these "aha" moments from your innovation network. It would be best to have a brain break for five minutes five times per day. This should be a time of zero effort, not to be confused with zero thought, because you're always thinking of something. So it's not enough to say, "Well, I'm going to shut down my brain. I'm not going to think about anything." That just doesn't work. It's about zero effort, not zero thought. Sometimes I will walk down the hall or outside at lunchtime. Other times I'll sit in my office and look out the window. These moments give my brain a chance to recharge. It's typically after I've completed a heavy-duty task, and I've gotten some completion and closure on that path. It may be after I've done two or three hours of meaningless emails.

When you go home after work, turn off the radio in your car. That'll be an experience. Don't focus on having an "aha" moment. Just drive without being distracted by the radio and see what that does for you in terms of recharging your brain.

Let's look at another example. You're an avid runner. While running, you stop at some point so your body can recharge and become relaxed. Maybe you lift weights. Well, you don't just keep on lifting forever. You have to stop for rest when your muscles tell you that your body needs a break. We've all been in meetings where we're working with other people on a project and think, "Man, I need a break." You can't use your brain all day long at its best without taking a break. You can, but you certainly won't achieve the desired results. You won't experience any "aha" moments. When a team of colleagues takes a break and reconvenes, someone usually pipes up, "While we were out, I thought of a new way we can tackle this."

Your brain is your best business weapon. You know more about your business than anybody. You know what works, what doesn't, and what your customers expect. So you have fixed knowledge about your business. But sometimes, that's the limit. Have you ever met somebody who can't see what they're doing in their business? I see this a lot.

Do you feel stuck doing the same thing over and over in your business? Once you learn how to use your brain effectively and develop a roadmap, you will start making progress. Sometimes you need an outside advisor to challenge your brain. But you can only do that if you have fine-tuned your brain to accept new information. So your brain is your best business weapon, and it's at your disposal daily.

It's also important to know that your brain never sleeps. You may be asleep, but your brain is still working. I think about it like a cleaning crew that comes into my brain each night to sweep out all of the partial ideas that aren't going anywhere. They organize my thinking and help me make sense of things I encountered during the day.

Implementing the three protocols of strategic attention by identifying elephants, limiting multitasking, and giving your brain opportunities to recharge will train your brain for optimal performance, leading to success in your professional and personal life.

KEY TAKEAWAYS

- Use the brainpower of two to prioritize two "to-do list" items per day that require strategy, analysis, and heavy-duty thinking. We refer to these tasks as "elephants."
- Aim to get these tasks done in 45 minutes, the amount of time your brain can focus entirely.
- "When you're hunting elephants, don't get distracted by chasing rabbits." Rabbits are mundane tasks that require little brain work

but often deter us from the elephant tasks that make us feel accomplished at the end of the day and move our needle forward.
- Remember that multitasking is doing two things at the same time with different goals.
- Chronic multitasking is toxic to your brain and leads to a decline in fluid intelligence.
- Use the brainpower of one to limit multitasking, sequence tasks one at a time, and eliminate distractions in your work environment.
- Use the brainpower of none to take brain breaks for five minutes five times per day. These breaks allow your brain to recharge and be more open to "aha" moments.

CHAPTER

3

BRAIN SCIENCE AND PERFORMANCE: INTEGRATED REASONING

Integrated reasoning involves setting a framework for heavy-duty problem-solving, planning, and strategizing. You've laid the foundation, closed the door, and eliminated as many distractions as possible. You've committed to doing one thing at a time, giving your brain the necessary breaks along the way. And now you're ready to do some real heavy-duty lifting and tackle those elephants in your life.

Strengthening networks occurs through the synthesis of information. We're bombarded with all kinds of information from various sources from the moment we wake up to the time we go to bed. We have to learn how to take some of it and throw it away because it's not of any value to us. Then we have to find the stuff that *is* important to us and synthesize that information so that when we're problem-solving, planning, or strategizing, we can make the best kinds of decisions. The great news is while we're doing this, we're strengthening our brains. We're building cognitive resources like weightlifting, which become available as we grow and attempt to accomplish other things.

THREE PROTOCOLS OF INTEGRATED REASONING

ZOOM IN

The first protocol of integrated reasoning is "zoom in," which is all about identifying critical information to achieve an in-depth understanding of the knowledge. What is critical information? If it's a business issue, critical information may have something to do with cost and benefit, and analysis. It also might be the availability of your time. That's an essential piece for understanding and resolving issues.

Many of us haven't learned how to be critical thinkers, and from time to time, I've gone through a day on autopilot of answering what I needed to answer. I've responded to emails and done some technical work but failed to identify an elephant. So the first step is to identify your elephant and really dig in; zoom in on all the critical information about the task.

In the following example, there will be a couple of errors that I will point out because it's important to understand that you don't live in a perfect world. And when you dig into the critical information about something, you may need to have a couple of different looks at it. You may have somebody else look at it. You should discuss something in depth because that's what it takes to have all the critical elements, such as money, time, resources, and relationships.

Let's say you lost your job and you need money fast. You go to Amazon, and they offer $18 an hour. They also tell you that you will drive your own car to make deliveries. You know that you need $30 an hour to maintain your lifestyle. So you have to do some analysis. Take a look at how many miles you are going to drive. The IRS says it costs 57 cents a mile or $114 daily. Let's say you work about six hours for Amazon. You want to make that $30 an hour or $180 total, but the cost to you is actually $294 when you factor in mileage and the wear and tear on your car. So it costs you to go to work. Some people might not see this initially because they get $18 an hour that wasn't in their pocket before.

Here's an error I want to point out. Let's say your car payment is $700 monthly, and gas is 30 cents a mile. So your cost for the day is not $114. It's the cost of the car *plus* the gas. So it's about $83 a day, and you still get that $18 an hour from Amazon. So you subtract your auto cost, and you're really making $4 an hour. Isn't that great? But you don't feel it because you have cash in your pocket to pay for the gas. Many people working for Amazon, Uber, or Lyft don't understand the financial impact on their vehicles.

As you can see, some information you analyze can be very technical and numbers oriented. And if you are looking at it yourself, it might look like it will work for you. Well, maybe it does for the short run, but it might not be such a great deal in the long run. So you have to take other things into account. What are the other things? How else could you spend your time? That's part of analyzing whether or not you want to drive for Amazon. What about your family? Can you spend more time with them? Do you have kids in school who need more attention to make sure they're achieving their goals? You could sit around and watch TV, but that's probably not a good use of your time. How about working out? If you feel better physically, you'll likely have higher motivation to get a better job. What is the impact on your vehicle and your body? Some people can't be in and out of a car all day long making deliveries.

Many people haven't developed the skills to look at scenarios so deeply. If I'm looking at taking on a client and doing work for them, I analyze the kind of work they'll require. I compare it to work that we do for other clients. I evaluate what they're asking for and whether they understand what they're getting from us for the price. I assess how they seem to be approaching the decision to hire a CPA firm. I analyze how they seem to react to new ideas and whether they're stuck. I explore whether they will want to take my time or if they're comfortable working with somebody I've trained and who can do the job as well.

All of these are examples of critical elements. Evaluating critical information is a skill, and it takes practice. Throughout my life, I've often just taken things at face value. And really, if you're going to use these tools, taking things at face value is a cop-out.

ZOOM OUT

The next step is to zoom out. That means taking this critical information you've zoomed in on and changing it to a more abstracted general idea.

Let's use a pricing example. You want to price your product. You think, "I'm going to deliver this product to my client, and this is how I'm going to price it." That's very narrow, and it's restrictive to you because that means you have to do that same thing for every client you deal with. Every time you sell that product or service, you must zoom in on it to that level.

The power of zooming out is to take this detailed information and make it into a generalized concept that says, overall, this is the way you're going to price and deliver your product. So you're taking a narrower picture and making it broader. It's transforming critical information into an abstracted generalized idea. Abstracted means you're not looking at this one single data point or this one single client, or this one single product. You're generalizing that into a broader picture. Solving the critical details of one incident doesn't apply to all the other places it might occur.

Remember that companies have gone through the zooming-out process when they arrive at a standardized price. They have analyzed individual client deliveries and figured out exactly what it takes. So they end up with an abstracted idea, zooming out from the particular client situation to a broader, generalized answer that can be applied to the entire company. It can be a change to the product or service, the same product or service delivered differently, or delivered by a different person. It could be a combination of products or services packaged as one unit. Ask yourself, "If it works this way for one client, how does it work for the company as a whole? How does it work in the marketplace? Will the market accept my definition of the product, pricing, and service the way I intended?"

ZOOM DEEP AND WIDE

The third and final step is to zoom deep and wide, which means creating new meaning. After discovering what your competitors are doing and zooming out to get a picture of that pricing model in the marketplace, you can create new meaning. Can you present it differently? Can you offer it with something else and change the context of delivering your product? It's a matter of combining your knowledge and experience with the details you discovered.

This is the legacy part of integrated reasoning because it applies personal context. So if you look at the pricing issue from a personal standpoint, you will say, "How does that affect me? Is it something

I can pull off? Do I have what it takes? Do I have other resources that would enable me to offer this up?" Looking at it from a personal context becomes a very in-depth view. It's not just, "Give me the facts and the big picture." It allows you to understand your relationship with the issue.

Let's say I want the absolute best product delivered by the most knowledgeable people. Well, that sounds really noble. In my business, that person would be me. And I only have 2,000 hours a year to spend at work because I do things outside of my work. So if I say it's got to be that way, I've created something that doesn't entirely solve the problem. A combination of other things solves the problem. Number one, training people in a way so that they can deliver the product or service effectively. Secondly, developing some technology and support around what we do. I'd be dead if I created a product or service that took me 3,000 hours a year to deliver. Why would I do that to myself? That tells me I've got to go beyond what I see as the critical data relating to a problem I'm solving or the growth I want to occur. I've got to go beyond just looking at how my company could deliver that work. I have to go to the personal level and determine that my needs are also met because I'm the primary owner of MindSmarts. So if I arrive at a great solution that might kill me in the process, it's not a very good solution. If I'm trying to grow MindSmarts, I have to look at what I bring to the table and what other people can bring to the table. I must begin applying my personal context to business decisions by combining my knowledge and experience with the problems I have encountered and am trying to solve.

With integrated reasoning, you can't continue to operate like a robot. You have to think, and thinking is hard work. If you're going to integrate this into your life and gain all the benefits from brain performance, you must start by identifying a roadmap. You develop the elephants every day that move you a step closer to what you're trying to accomplish. And each step of the way, you dig into it. The more you zoom in, zoom out, and zoom deep and wide to get a complete picture, the more you can make good decisions and create new meaning. This can be very exciting. If you're solving a problem in your company that's been keeping you up at night, this is an excellent way to grow your business and do something you've never done before.

Don't forget; your brain loves to work hard. If you're going through the motions, it causes brain atrophy and slows your brain plasticity. But higher-order thinking grows your brain as you participate in heavy-duty analysis, planning, implementing, and applying knowledge.

KEY TAKEAWAYS

- Synthesizing important information strengthens the brain and leads to better decision-making.
- Integrated reasoning consists of three protocols: zoom in, zoom out, and zoom deep and wide.
- Zoom in to identify critical information to achieve an in-depth understanding of the knowledge. Evaluating critical information takes skill and practice.
- Zoom out to take critical information you've zoomed in on and change it to a more abstracted general idea that will work for multiple clients and the marketplace.
- Zoom deep and wide to create new meaning and apply personal context to business decisions.

CHAPTER 4

BRAIN SCIENCE AND PERFORMANCE: INNOVATION

Innovation, the third set of brain training protocols, is defined as enhancing performance through flexible thinking. When we hear "innovation," we think about people like Jeff Bezos and Richard Branson, racing their rockets to outer space, or Elon Musk, who created the Tesla. Sometimes you might feel you need more resources, knowledge, or millions of dollars to innovate. But innovation as it relates to you and your business can be tiny.

We talked about how brain training is similar to a physical workout, building endurance to think clearly, creatively, and deeply about things that matter to you. Then we discussed integrated reasoning and zooming in, zoning out, and zooming deep and wide to develop strategic long-term solutions or application of new knowledge to old problems, so you can begin to think transitionally instead of transactionally. Being innovative is about flexibility and not getting trapped in an old way of thinking.

So what does innovation mean? Is it what Elon Musk does? Well, sure, he's innovative. What about those Silicon Valley people who have created all kinds of products? Yeah, certainly.

What about Apple? Apple is interesting. Apple was almost out of business shortly after it started. Apple's goal was to compete with Microsoft, which dominated 85% to 90% of the small computer environment of the world. If Apple continued to compete in only that realm, it wouldn't exist today. Why were they successful? They went back and looked at what business they *really* needed to be in. It was really about storing personal information. That's their business now, which includes the iPhone and the cloud. They could only compete with Microsoft once they changed what they envisioned as their future. That's innovation.

So innovation is more than being able to come up with something as big as Amazon, developing the next app, or becoming Jeff Bezos. ***It's a continuous pursuit of original thinking to build new value, meaning, or knowledge and shape the future.*** If you constantly pursue original thinking to build new value about what you deliver to people, new meaning or knowledge to how it can be applied, and you're trying to shape the future, then, congratulations, you're being innovative. Innovation may mean taking some product from somebody else, altering it, giving it a new value, adding to it, changing the meaning of how it's used, and using your knowledge to end up with something different that you offer to clients.

We're in a service-oriented society much more than we used to be in a manufacturing society. As a service provider, myself as a CPA, it's essential to look at things differently, try to be original, and add new value. This can apply to your product offerings or how you educate clients and staff. It is not only you; innovation also applies to employees. Perhaps your staff is stuck in the back corner of floor

14 of your office building; they can be innovative by identifying new ways to serve your clients and even create new value in a way to service all your clients and add new meaning and value to the services your company offers…to shape the future of the business.

THE THREE BRAINPOWERS OF INNOVATION

1. **Brainpower of Infinite:** Recognize that there are an infinite number of alternative ways to solve your business problems. Identify multiple solutions and discover limitless ways to attack a problem by appreciating various perspectives.
2. **Brainpower of Paradox:** Recognize that making mistakes creates the most fertile ground for growth. I've always thought of mistakes as opportunities rather than problems. And I've got gray hair, so I've made plenty of mistakes. I've made people angry, I've been fired, and I've misread situations. But I'm still here. The brainpower of paradox is about reflecting and reframing to maximize the opportunity to learn and apply something new.
3. **Brainpower of the Unknown:** Create a cultivated position of curiosity, encouraging you to be a change creator, not a change blocker. MindSmarts has resulted in a significant change to my CPA firm. It's a recognition that the last thing we do in the business cycle is a tax return and financial statements for our clients. Before that, the clients make business decisions, implement processes, come up with financial results, and hopefully earn enough cash and profits to pay their taxes. It's pretty destabilizing to think that, as CPAs, we really should be at the front end of that process, helping

our clients make better business decisions from the very start. We shouldn't just be at the back end doing tax returns. We'll continue to do them since it's part of our service, but it's innovative on our part to offer High-Performance Brain Training to improve business performance earlier in the business decision cycle.

YOUR LIZARD BRAIN

How's your lizard brain doing these days? Did you even know you had a lizard brain? Have you named yours? The name of my lizard brain is Remington. Before you start thinking I've gone crazy, let's define what a lizard brain is. Lizard brain refers to how you act when you encounter something threatening, such as a new idea, new boss, new concept at work, or a date with someone new. There's an initial response when you encounter something fearful, also known as fight or flight. So when a cat or a dog is threatening a lizard, it's not just pondering on the rock; it's getting ready to run. Your amygdala is the gut-level emotional response portion of your brain. So when you first encounter something that's threatening to you, your amygdala kicks in.

We've all experienced this. When I first got in front of a camera, my amygdala kicked in because I had no clue about this camera stuff. When this happens, you must have a way to change how you look at the situation because otherwise, you will take off running.

The solution lies in activating your frontal lobe. We've discussed various training techniques and methods to grow your frontal lobe. So the first thing you do is step back and focus on the bigger picture. It's your logical, executive brain that's working for you here. Then you start balancing things, figuring out the new scenario's upsides and downsides. For example, let's say you have a new boss. What's the upside? Maybe they will like you, give you more responsibility, or use your talents more effectively. On the downside, they may determine you need to do a better job.

Perhaps you have a client who decides to leave your firm or buy their product elsewhere. What does that mean? On the upside, maybe the client was hard to deal with, and it now allows you to deal with more clients better suited to you. On the downside, this may be the start of many clients following suit and leaving.

After you've balanced the scale, you engage in possibility thinking, which is part of the brainpower of infinite. Look at all the possible solutions to solve the problem at hand. You're being innovative at that point. You're saying, "Well, what are all the possibilities? Maybe that means a great opportunity for us to do something differently." Open your mind to the many possible solutions. Your frontal lobe will take over, and the executive network will determine the best course of action. This is how you make the switch from your lizard brain.

Many business owners don't want to admit they're afraid of anything. I know I don't. But my lizard brain Remington is there to tell me that I need to look out for something. So then I implement these switches. I go into my frontal lobe first, being neutral, balancing the pluses and minuses, seeking all the possible alternatives, and then making a decision. You can do that too. Innovation begins when you can switch from a lizard brain to a Jeff Bezos brain.

IMPLEMENTING TACTILE SWITCHES

The following business scenario will teach you how to engage those tactical switches during challenging times. I'm a CPA, so let's say a client fires me. That doesn't feel good. I like to provide excellent service and make people feel like they are getting value. I want them to know we work hard on their behalf. So if somebody were to fire me, it would be upsetting no matter who it was.

The first thing I would do is zoom out to see the bigger picture. What kind of client is this? Is it my largest client? Is it a once-a-year tax return? Is there a deeper issue? Was it something I did or something my firm did? So I step out to see the bigger picture and put it in perspective. Then I say, "Well, there are infinite possibilities. Some positive, some negative." Was this client an ideal client? Is it someone I would want to work with again? Everybody should have a picture of their ideal customer or client, which will help with this analysis. If they weren't a perfect client, it could be positive that they're gone. Another positive is that this could be a wake-up call regarding how my firm served the client. Perhaps they weren't even a financially significant client or didn't have much growth possibility…more positives.

Then I would examine the negatives. Am I doing a poor job of serving all my clients? What if this were a major client? What would it have done to the company? After balancing the positives and negatives, I move on to the brainpower of paradox, examining actions I have taken in the past and determining how they relate to this case. For example, years ago, I had a major client; as they grew, they outgrew my small accounting firm for a larger one. Their accounting fees went up dramatically. But my fees went down to

$0 for that particular client. What did I learn? I learned that my firm would survive because I view life and business as a vacuum. Something always comes back to fill in the void. There will always be new clients or more work for existing clients. So when I look at the brainpower of paradox, I realize that losing a significant client may hurt for a while, but we end up coming back even stronger.

What about the brainpower of the unknown? Remember that you can not always know the outcome of any decision; the outcome is unknown until you try some solution. Looking back, should I do things the same way I have done in the past or change them up? There are many options to solve a negative problem like losing a client. But let's spin it to a more positive problem. Let's say you have the opportunity to pick up a big client comprising 10% of your revenue, but you don't have all the staff you need to serve this client. Using the same techniques, you could be fearful of taking on a client that big, but on the other hand, you can find innovative ways to serve that client. If you turn to your executive network and frontal lobe, you can determine the best course of action and implementation. Remember that implementing, planning, and strategizing for something like this is the best use of your brain. It grows your brain capacity, white matter, and blood flow as you grow your cognitive resources. As a result, all ships rise, and you improve your cognitive ability, social interaction, business problem-solving, resilience, daily life, and quality of life. So when you consider innovation, think about applying it to anything your company is facing. Use the brainpowers of infinite, paradox, or unknown to examine things differently. Be a change-maker for your company.

CHALLENGE YOUR INNOVATIVE THINKING

One way to encourage creative thinking is to devise an analogy of what it's like to do your job daily. For example, doing my job is like being a giraffe. I have to look up high and all around to find the best leaves on the tree. Even though I'm down in the depths of tax returns and financial statements, I have to look high and broad. So that's an analogy. Creating analogies makes you use your brain powerfully and think about things differently.

Perhaps you do your job like a wise old owl sitting on a perch, pontificating the positives and negatives of various scenarios. Or maybe you're like a squirrel running from here to there and back and forth from one task to another. Generating analogies to talk about what you do is being innovative.

Think about three ways you've been innovative in the last 30 days. I can think about ways that I've been innovative, and a couple of them have been related to MindSmarts; one was tweaking something to ensure our clients are getting what they bargained for in the form of a survey questionnaire after they work with us. It was innovative because we hadn't used this kind of tool before.

Are there places this last week or this coming week that would serve you to be more flexible? Can you go into your workweek with some unusual way of looking at things and be open to accepting somebody else's ideas? Can you seek new ideas that will give you mental flexibility so you have some responsibility for using all these protocols? It is your responsibility to use them.

Some people are stuck in how they view the world and won't think much about the concept of brain training, while others will realize the tremendous value of MindSmarts. That's what innovation is all about. It's not for everyone. But MindSmarts is about continuously pursuing original thinking and building new value, meaning, or knowledge to shape the future.

KEY TAKEAWAYS

- Innovation enhances performance through flexible thinking. It is the continuous pursuit of original thinking to build new value, meaning, or knowledge and shape the future.
- The brainpower of infinite allows us to identify multiple solutions and discover limitless ways to attack a problem by appreciating various perspectives.
- The brainpower of paradox is about reflecting and reframing to maximize the opportunity to learn something new, often due to an error or mistake.
- The brainpower of the unknown creates a cultivated position of curiosity, encouraging us to be change creators, not change blockers, even though the result will be unknown until we try it.
- Learn to switch from a "lizard brain" to a "Jeff Bezos" brain to avoid running from perceived threats, new challenges, and novel ideas.
- Engage tactical switches and the three brainpowers to examine problems your company is facing differently.
- Create analogies to challenge your innovative thinking and use your mind powerfully.

CHAPTER 5

ROADMAP

Former New York Yankee Manager Yogi Berra once said, "If you don't know where you are going, you will end up somewhere else!" Even with a destination in mind, you still need a map. A roadmap will show you how to get where you want to go. Without a map, you may end up anywhere. And in some cases, that's okay. A friend of mine once told me, "All those who wander are not lost; they just lack clarity."

There was a time in my life when I had a lot of serious, comprehensive goals. I had goals related to work, health, romance, travel, education, having children, and housing. I looked at these goals every day. They were specific; they were measurable; they were achievable. They were realistic and time-based, but even so, having goals didn't work for me.

There were other times in my life when I had no goals. I had a great job, and I was achieving things in my career. I had a good income; I was living a comfortable life for my age and level of life experience. I didn't squander money or possess a voracious appetite for spending. So I had what I needed to live my life. But I didn't have a clear picture of where I was going because I relied on my ability to be productive and efficient and attempted to become a better performer. Having substantial goals in my life didn't help or hinder me, nor did having no goals. I'm a productive kind of person either way. So sometimes, people who don't have goals can accomplish far more than somebody who has self-limiting goals.

Think about this: If your goal is to make $100,000 and you reach $101,000, you'll feel like you did a great job. But the reality is, if you didn't have a goal, maybe you could have made a million dollars. Sometimes goals can be limiting, and people respond differently to them. Some respond well to "quality of life" goals, and others to "quantity" goals. Some people respond to goals that lead to other goals, such as, "If I accomplish X, then I can do Y." Some set goals compared to last year, which is a pretty poor way to go about it, but that's what many people do. Why is that the case?

Let's say you have a small company with revenues of $300,000 a year, and you're surviving on the profits. You say, "Okay, I want a million in sales next year. My profit goal is $200,000. I'm only going to work 40 hours a week and want a nice vacation." So what's wrong with that? The goals may be okay, but there's nothing to tell you how to get there. There needs to be a roadmap or strategy. Otherwise, it's just a number. So sometimes, having a goal sounds great. But what are you doing to reach that goal? It would be best if you had a plan.

Perhaps you did better than last year on sales. Somebody might say, "Hey, that's excellent!" But instead of focusing on doing better than last year, you should focus on achieving something based on specific plans.

I'm not saying goals are bad, especially if they make you ask better questions. It's also possible to set goals that are much too aggressive. Maybe your goal is to reach $10 million and live on the beach in Tahiti next year. That's a bad goal without a plan to get there in a year. But bad goals make you ask good questions. What were you planning to do if you didn't make $10 million? Were you planning to live off existing customers and hope they grow? Were you planning to hire a salesforce? Do you have a marketing system in place to give you leads? So it's okay to have a less-than-stellar goal as long as it forces you to ask the right questions.

ROADMAP VS. GOAL

I aim to educate people about brain health and performance and use High-Performance Brain Training protocols in business. It's a great goal, but it's only a destination, and it's nothing without a plan, or a roadmap, to get there.

Goals are very concrete and specific. "I want to do $10 million in business by 2025. I want to hire three people. I want to go from Dallas to Seattle." Generally, goals are also measurable. If your goal is to do $10 million in revenue and you've only reached $1 million, that's measurable. Roadmaps are also measurable, but not in such an unbending way. Each strategic step can be specific, concrete, and measurable, but a roadmap allows flexibility to recover from problems as you follow your road. For example, I wanted this chapter to be done a week ago, but due to other things, I couldn't accomplish that. I'm still getting it done now, but my roadmap gave me the flexibility to do so.

As business owners, we always want to have goals for our business. But that's not enough. You must have a plan to hold yourself accountable for the end destination and all the steps you must take to get there. It's about asking the "how" questions. "How will I accomplish this? How will I handle the situation if X, Y, or Z happens?"

Keep in mind, as business owners; we also have personal lives. Your identity is so wrapped up in your business that your roadmap will inevitably include items from your personal life. You get to decide the balance between your personal and business life, which will be unique for everyone. A complete roadmap includes your personal life, as it is challenging to do something personal without thinking about how it will ultimately affect the business and vice versa.

You might think, "What happens if I veer off course?" Covid threw everyone off course. Business owners were forced to adapt to new ways of doing things. With the knowledge you now have on High-Performance Brain Training, you would have had the skills to be innovative in the challenging Covid times and today as well. People were working from home or no longer working at all. Life looked totally different for many. So even when dealing with a roadmap, it's essential to be honest about your goals and give yourself grace if you don't reach them.

Think about a goal you didn't reach. It might have been due to a lack of a roadmap. What if your goal was to reach $1 million in sales this year, and it didn't happen? Did you plan for the sales effort? Did you have enough leads? Did you produce the product efficiently? Those roadmap pieces may have needed to be added to your original plan.

"WHAT? SO WHAT? NOW WHAT?"

It's essential to make your goals personal to increase your chances of success. Examine your roadmap with the following questions in mind, "What? So what? Now what?" The "what" is your end target, whether immediate or long-term. Let's say it's to make a million dollars. So what? Why do you want to make a million dollars? How would that impact your life? The truth is, many small businesses are doing a million dollars in sales. My firm does, but what does that mean to my employees and me? How does it influence our opportunities and standards? Understand how rich and meaningful the goal is to your life so that you can move on to the final step, "What next?" What will you do tomorrow to get closer to that target?

This is a test. Does "What? So what? Now what?" sound familiar? This is another way to talk about integrated reasoning: zooming in, zooming out, and zooming deep and wide. When thinking about your roadmap or any other business chapter in this book, use the knowledge of High-Performance Brain Training to apply these protocols to your business problems, opportunities, and solutions.

TIMEFRAMES

Almost every target or goal has a timeframe. Long-term goals require a different kind of strategic thinking. If you're saving for a down payment for a home, you can't do that overnight; it might take three years. If you want to reach a million in sales, it might happen next year if you implement the right strategies, but if you don't, it could take two or three years.

We have all had the experience of sitting around the dinner table in mid-September and saying, "Where did the year go? It's almost Christmas!" When we have these kinds of feelings, we aren't relating them to the timeframe of our roadmap. Regarding roadmap timeframes, I recommend three-year, one-year, and 90-day timeframes.

Why? We can generally relate to some life event within a three-year timeframe. For example, your oldest may be out of high school, you will be settled in your new house, or you will have worked out product delivery and profitability in your business.

Next comes one-year goals. If you know your target for three years, and a year has passed, you know that you need to get moving if you are not a third of the way through your progress. So let's say you're starting a business. You should define the product or service in the first year. In year two, you want to establish more permanent operations and quit your job. You might envision the business fully supporting your family in the third year. All of those are very aggressive goals, so you must act strategically.

If you think about a one-year cycle, it's easier to forecast technology, marketing, staffing, and even anomalies like Covid. But that one-year forecast isn't enough. The real keys are the 90-day sprints. What will you do Monday morning to help you reach your goals strategically? The 90-day work propels you forward and allows you to gain confidence in completing activities on the highway of your roadmap. You can begin to identify other needed resources such as people, marketing systems, and lead generation programs. You can also use 90-day sprints to evaluate whether your three-year and one-year targets are valid.

Let's look at what you might do in your first 90-day sprint when you start a business. Determine your product or service, give it a name, develop a marketing strategy, identify your ideal customer, run your business plan by others, and map out the financials with a CPA and attorney. Not having a concrete 90-day sprint might delay your business start by months, even years.

In the second 90-day sprint, you develop some agility and

standardization. Suppose you didn't accomplish everything in the first 90 days. Evaluate why and implement those items in this second sprint. Sometimes, it's as simple as forgetting to celebrate results.

It's essential to review financial statements every 90 days. Everything you do in business has a financial impact. The bottom line determines whether you have enough money to reinvest back into the business, live on, and pay Uncle Sam.

Remember that there are more to 90-day sprints than just the routine stuff. Special topics should also be covered, including whether your business is ready to sell. How attractive is it to others? How dependent is the business on you? What will you do after you sell the business? Business owners sometimes need to remember to make these considerations an early part of the roadmap. Whether your end goal is to build the business value so you can retire comfortably, to have a business to pass on to your kids or to change the world, it starts with your first 90-day sprint.

If you go any further out into the future with your goals, it's more likely things will change, and it makes it too easy to give yourself an excuse. The further out your goals are, the more difficult it is to be specific about them. Ten-year goals are important but will be less specific by their very nature. How do you measure these types of legacy plans? Perhaps you want to be a leader in your industry in ten years. Will that be based on your sales? Or participation in industry meetings and groups? Will it be based on the number of people you hire or the size of your customer base? As you can see, assessing and measuring long-term goals is much more challenging.

PUT IT ON PAPER

One of the most important parts of having a roadmap is to put it on paper. If you don't have it written down, it's easy to make excuses because you don't have clarity. And it's tough to force yourself into clarity unless you have it right in front of you. In my case, as I tried to complete content videos for MindSmarts.com, it helped to have my written 90-day sprint staring me in the face.

You can use whatever format you prefer for your roadmap, whether a pad of paper, Excel spreadsheet, or Word document, as long as it includes three-year targets, one-year targets, and 90-day sprints. After you complete the first 90-day sprint, you can create a second one separately. These 90-day sprints keep you honest. Keep in mind; bad goals are better than no goals. Bad goals are reasonable because they still force you to ask questions.

When you put your first roadmap together, commit time to it. Don't be surprised if it takes you an entire day or longer. This isn't something to toy with. It's the strategic life of your business. You have the tools of strategic attention, integrated reasoning, and innovation to be successful at this important task. Think carefully and take the time to make it very specific so that you know what to do tomorrow morning, on the first day of the 90-day sprint.

COACH OR DIY?

Do you really need a coach or business advisor? Many people think they can do it themselves. Don't get me wrong; some people do an excellent job. We live in a "DIY" world. But why do you think professions like life coaches and psychologists (and CPAs, for that matter) exist? People need an outside perspective to make sense of their lives and clarify their goals. Business owners tend to be DIY people, but they might need a coach to take advantage of some necessary benefits.

Sure, doing it yourself takes less time (so you think). You can go to Google and ask a question. It will take less time than meeting with someone and listening to their ideas. You can find information on process management, pricing, and cash flow to help determine if you are doing things correctly. It's also less expensive (so you think). Knowledge isn't free; an advisor will charge you for their services. Most business owners have a high level of self-trust in their knowledge and experience, or they wouldn't have gone into business in the first place.

But let's pause for a second. How reliable is Google? Do you ever see ads that say, "Our product is amazing, but don't expect us to tell you the shortfalls?" How about, "There was an independent study that showed our company to be the fourth worst in the industry?" or "Hey, you don't have to buy from us because you can go to _____ and get it for free?" Of course not. Google can be highly misleading and great at avoiding giving you the information you need to make informed decisions. I read that Google has eliminated 3.4 billion false ads; did you rely on any of those?

So doing it yourself only saves you time if you don't end up going down rabbit holes and trying things that are not focused on getting what you really need. People that advertise on Google aren't stupid. They know their product and will undoubtedly present it in a perfect light. How often do you go past page one or two of your Google result search? You always end up on page one through advertising or SEO, making it appear like that particular result is the only or best answer. But there may be 5,000 other pages with greater detail and vital information.

For example, let's say you want an LLC. You go to LegalZoom.com and pop in there to form an entity. Do you really understand what you did? What about the tax consequences of a franchise tax versus income tax? In the long run, you will spend more on penalties than you would have if you hired a professional to help you set things up correctly.

Business owners often feel that "it's lonely at the top" when they are the only ones making the tough decisions. You're getting demands from employees, customers, and vendors. You're thinking about financing, you've got cash flow issues, and your taxes might be due. You need to strategize for new products. Sometimes it's not lonely at the top; it's just too congested. There's too much going on in your brain at one time.

And sometimes, you need someone else to discuss those issues with and run your solutions by, even if you don't want to admit it. It would be best if you had someone else to hold you accountable. You may be knowledgeable in one area and not so much in another. It's a strength to ask someone else to help you in those areas and hold you accountable. Asking questions is a strength; it's not a weakness because gaining clarity and answers improves you and your decision-making. If you need to know what tools are available, it's an excellent time to consult with a coach or an advisor. Consultants are typically specific implementers for processes at your company (think software). Coaches and advisors provide vision and strategy for the overall direction of your business.

Now that you've been given the foundation to build a successful roadmap, I encourage you to create your first one. Remember that a roadmap consists of strategic activities to reach your destination. Lack of focus has killed far more businesses than lack of capital.

KEY TAKEAWAYS

- A goal is only a destination. It requires a roadmap of strategic activities to get there.
- Goals are never "bad" if they force you to ask good questions.
- A roadmap should always include your business and personal life in the components of three-year targets, one-year targets, and 90-day sprints.
- Long-term goals are reasonable to have but more challenging to measure; that is why you need 90-day sprints.
- Make goals personal to increase your chances of success, asking, "What? So what? Now what?"
- Put your roadmap on paper because the clarity right in front of you is hard to ignore.
- Seeking out knowledge from coaches and advisors is a strength, not a weakness; it costs less time and money in the long run and can provide vision and strategy for your roadmap.

CHAPTER 6

PRICING YOUR PRODUCT

There are three ways that business owners generally go about pricing their products, requiring varying levels of deep thinking and innovation, or sometimes, none at all.

1. **What the Market Will Bear:** This short-term strategy doesn't involve understanding the customer, resulting in customer turnover and erratic pricing. The only thinking that occurs is guessing at what a maximum price might be.
2. **My Competition Sets the Price:** This is another strategy that lacks deep thinking and empathy for the customer. It does not distinguish you as a business owner from anyone else. Using this method, you are choosing to be a commodity and not using the powers the brain wants and deserves to grow, including analysis, planning, deciding, measuring, and evaluating. To get out of this mindset, you must be honest about what you offer and why it differs from your competition. Give your process a name and even trademark

it. Communicate the uniqueness of this process to your prospects, and then deliver on it!
3. **My Costs Set the Price:** This method requires deep thinking protocols in integrated reasoning and allows an owner to be innovative when setting the price. The real issue is not only cost but volume. If your rent is $100K, your labor is $100K, and you can produce 1,000 units of time or product, the cost is $200 per unit. But what is your cost if the volume falls to 500 units? That's right; it becomes $400 per unit.

The analysis of cost and volume requires deep thinking protocols. **Zoom in** to the costs and the volume that can be produced, and **zoom out** to examine themes within the pricing. Are you a market leader in price or a low-cost leader? Are you priced higher because you want to be known as a quality leader? Finally, **zoom deep and wide** to make it personal and determine what kind of business owner you want to be remembered as.

This analysis also includes the innovation protocols. The **brainpower of infinite** refers to the endless possibilities to arrive at cost estimates, volume estimates, and other variables such as value pricing and subscription. The **brainpower of paradox** requires the owner to realize that "nothing is a given." If a mistake is made in any pricing elements, the owner can recover from this mistake and build resilience. The **brainpower of the unknown** is simply understanding you can't know the answer beforehand. You must make a decision and evolve as more information becomes available from the real world over time. This broadens the equation to include dissecting costs into variable and fixed (don't be afraid to talk to your CPA). It also includes understanding who your client is, what type of marketing you need to reach sales of 1,000 units, and planning the labor force necessary to produce goods and services. Overall, it requires an investment of time into planning.

There can be complex reasoning involved regarding costs, bringing us to the dreaded word "accounting," which most people don't like or understand. But you often don't have to use complex computations to understand essential concepts. For example, integrated reasoning is beneficial even if you don't understand everything and get the correct answer right off the bat. Why? Using integrated reasoning increases the blood flow to your brain, growing your white matter, which acts as the highway between your frontal lobe and amygdala. The amygdala houses your memory and emotional center. Brain growth from integrated reasoning has been proven by over 600 clinical studies from over 100 neuroscientists from the Center for BrainHealth.

PRICING IN THE REAL WORLD

Let's look at how integrated reasoning made Frito-Lay a wildly successful company. Years ago, they introduced bean dip; it was highly profitable at a sales price of $.17 per can. Despite the high-profit margin and the excellent taste, it just didn't sell. After some diligent market research, they learned that the low price actually discouraged customers from serving the product to their friends for fear of it not being "good enough." So what did Frito-Lay do? They raised the price to $.35, and it flew off the shelves! Zooming out allowed Frito-Lay to see what their customers were seeing. They dramatically improved profits by selling the bean dip based on costs and customer desires.

Next, let's look at how zooming in can be applied to pricing in today's marketplace. Zooming in is about understanding all the elements that make up your costs and examining them in great depth. For example, delivery costs could be one of those elements. When zooming in on delivery costs, consider questions like: Are you delivering? Is FedEx or UPS delivering? Are you combining multiple products in deliveries? How will you match customer time requirements to the delivery method? Delivery costs are significant because they can be more than the cost of making your product. Please zoom in to understand that even with a service business, the time to deliver the result and discuss it with the customer can be costly.

How can we use **all** brain training protocols to tackle the delivery cost topic? Besides zooming in, you can use the brainpower of infinite to open your mind to other delivery methods you have never considered. While doing this, incorporate the brainpower of one to nurture quiet contemplation without interruption. Don't forget the power of paradox to remind you that the world won't end if you make the wrong choice. Lastly, the definition of "innovation" is the constant striving to bring new meaning to your world. For example, Domino's Pizza gives a $3 discount on the next order to customers who pick up their own pizzas for their current order. How innovative! They already encouraged customers to order again and solved their delivery problem simultaneously. That's an excellent way to be innovative amongst other restaurants that only focus on deliveries!

In the examples above, we zoomed in and out, but what about zooming deep and wide? I define this as the "legacy" protocol because it makes the decision personal to you. You begin thinking about themes and give life to these themes by making them personal. For example, if you decide to use a subscription pricing model, will this model change what is delivered to your clients? How will your customers view you? Will they see you as trying to make a buck or giving them more for their dollar? How do you consider yourself using this model? Are you modernizing your service? Are you adding value? Are you gaining efficiency that will help you and your clients? Does this model provide something to build on for future success? If choosing this method gives you a personal identity that serves you, it becomes your legacy.

If you choose the same subscription model and don't go through the complete range of protocols, you may accept the choice but not "buy into it" completely. You won't have a solid understanding of the full scope of the benefits and issues related to the choice. Because of this, you may not follow the model entirely and, as a result, have too many exceptions, inefficiencies, confused clients, and annoyed staff.

Pricing is complex for most companies because they don't really understand what their customers are buying; on top of that, they don't understand their costs; even then, they are inconsistent in applying the costs. How can a company owner know which products are more profitable if inconsistent? Couple this inconsistency with accounting systems that don't measure costs by product or revenue stream, and the resulting analysis of cost and profit will be sketchy. When you decide to take on a totally new pricing method, you will incorporate all of the integrated reasoning and innovation tools to consider the full scope of information needed to get the most robust and complete answer.

As a final note, review the brainpower of paradox and the brainpower of the unknown. As you decide on a pricing strategy for your services, consider the possibility that the results of your decisions are unknown until you test them in the marketplace. Consider also that the market may reject your pricing. What is the worst that can happen? You may lose a customer opportunity and have to go back to choose another pricing model. There are no givens when it comes to pricing except that customers buy because they want and desire what you provide. The price is only part of it. However, pricing is complex because of all these issues. Continue to apply the integrated reasoning strategies to customer responses to your pricing. The customer that won't buy from you under your pricing model may be like all other prospects, or they might be the *only* one who tells you why.

KEY TAKEAWAYS

- Use the "My Costs Sets the Price" method to analyze cost and volume using deep thinking protocols and innovation.
- Integrated reasoning increases blood flow to your brain, growing your white matter because you feed the brain what it craves…analyzing, measuring, evaluating, comparing, planning, innovating, and deep thinking.
- Incorporate all of the integrated reasoning and innovation tools to arrive at pricing that satisfies your customers and leaves a desirable legacy for your business.

CHAPTER 7

CASH FLOW

What in the world is cash flow? And why is it such a problem for many small businesses? Everything from the start of a business until it closes its doors relates to cash. It is almost impossible to begin a business without some cash in your pocket. Typically, you take some savings (cash) or borrow (cash) and form your organization. Then you spend cash to find customers (marketing) and convince them to buy from you (sales). Then you need to work to deliver through your own efforts or an employee or contractor. Even if you have a client ready to buy from you, you have the costs of organization and other start-up costs that require cash.

Throughout the life of your business, you will make profits, borrow money, bill and collect, buy assets, acquire expenses, pay taxes, and finally, pay yourself. When you get ready to close down the business, you will sell off the assets, pay the bills, and take whatever cash is left. Cash is a cradle-to-grave concept. Between the start and the end, you will do a lot of work that doesn't affect cash immediately; you must manage the timing of the business functions with the receipt or expenditure of cash. The timing of cash causes most of the cash flow problems for business owners. However, cash flow problems are typically the RESULT of other problems, not the CAUSE.

The difference between the success or failure of a business may be how they use cash. I will sound like your Grandpa, "Live on less than you make," "Save something out of every dollar you make." If you do those things, you have a leg up on the business down the street that is always short of cash and on the edge of bankruptcy.

From a High-Performance Brain Training perspective, I realized that many small business owners think short-term and are not strategic in their business decisions. As you know, I refer to this as the "Trapped Business Owner" syndrome. The recognition of this short-term thinking took me to the Center for BrainHealth in 2019 to learn whether their High-Performance Brain Training protocols could help business owners become more long-term and strategic in their thinking. The science from over 600 clinical studies shows that this is the case.

Even though short-term thinking affects every area of business, it most commonly relates to cash flow. You will learn that cash flow problems result from other issues brought on by short-term thinking. Throughout this chapter on cash flow, you will be encouraged to utilize the High-Performance Brain Training protocols to become more strategic in your business. Being more strategic will help you recognize and address the underlying issues that are showing up in your cash flow.

Short-term thinking puts a business in panic mode. It isn't easy to become strategic when the reality is that you need enough cash to make payroll on Friday. So set the stage for your transition to thinking more strategically and long-term by implementing the protocols in strategic attention.

STRATEGIC ATTENTION AND CASH FLOW

First, apply your thinking to just one thing at a time. You have learned that multitasking is toxic to your brain; humans are not wired to do two things simultaneously. Close the door, turn off the radio, and hold your calls. Then identify two elephants daily that will move your needle forward professionally or personally.

Start with an elephant that gets you in touch with who your customer is and why they became a customer. Your understanding of your customer will be a foundational part of your strategic thinking. Aim to complete this elephant in 45 minutes. Do you remember why? Your brain can only focus for 45 minutes before becoming distracted. This being the case, you may have to break down your analysis of your customer into several sections before you have a complete understanding. This alone may take you several weeks to complete.

Finally, give your brain a break. If you are operating in anxiety or panic mode to meet short-term obligations, your brain is tired. Take a break and let your brain find solutions for you.

WHAT IS CASH FLOW MANAGEMENT?

Remember that customer who was ready to buy from you before you started your business? He said, "Bill me when complete." If it takes you a month to complete the work and the worker is you,

you need to get paid, don't you? The month ends, and you bill this new customer, but he doesn't pay you immediately. He pays you the following month. By that time, you've had to pay yourself for two months while incurring multiple other costs of running a business. And if you don't have enough cash to cover those costs and payroll, you forgo your own paycheck. And then the cycle begins again, not leaving you very much money to grow your business. It's easy to get stuck with nowhere to go.

Without cash, you can't invest in equipment, marketing, personnel, and all the other necessary growth components. Businesses often make up for this lack of cash by bootstrapping, basically making do with what little resources they have, including their own energy. The Oxford definition of bootstrapping is to "get (oneself or something) into or out of a situation using existing resources." If you rely on resources from third parties, investors, or lenders, you are not bootstrapping.

Bootstrapping creates all types of good habits that will help a business survive. In fact, it is often a bad idea to have all the cash you need at the start. With excess cash, it is easy to overspend and blow through it without having developed the cash management tools to handle it wisely. Bootstrapping is a great place to use the innovation protocols of High-Performance Brain Training. If you seek ways to use minimal resources (cash, for example) to accomplish things, you need to be innovative. Remember the definition of innovation: "A continuous pursuit of original thinking to build new value, meaning, knowledge and shape the future." Can you think of a more important place to use this set of Brain Performance tools?

There are many functions in a business that happen without cash; customers and vendors who don't pay you right away, inventory that needs to be pre-purchased and kept on hand, purchasing equipment, and hiring employees. You will spend a lot of cash before you start seeing profits. It's all about timing. It would be best if you managed the timing of credit before it turns into cash. You give credit and receive credit. It is a well-known axiom that if you want to grow your business, offer more accessible credit. If you make it easy for someone to buy through volume discounts and excellent terms, you will be able to sell more. However, with higher sales, you need cash to do the work before the customer payments come in. Where will you get the cash you need? You can borrow from a bank, getting cash in exchange for bank credit. At some point, the bank will need to be paid back. Hopefully, all your customers will pay, and you will have the cash you need. If you manage your cash flow, you will have the funds. If you don't, you won't. It's as simple as that.

THE OBJECTIVES OF CASH FLOW: SPEED UP OR SLOW DOWN THE FLOW

In understanding the elements of cash flow management, you can use the integrated reasoning protocols of zooming in, zooming out, and zooming deep and wide. Zooming in will lead you to deep thinking about the detailed elements affecting cash flow. Zooming out will allow you to see the themes behind the cash flow issues, such as setting expectations for customer payment terms or the speed at which you find qualified prospects and convert them to customers. Zooming deep and wide might lead you to contemplate how you want to run your business. Do you always want to be short of cash and fight this battle forever? Or do you want to manage the cash flow so it works for you, not against you?

The objective of cash flow management is to have enough cash when you need it to pay your monthly expenses and accumulate cash for reinvesting in your business and making a profit, all while balancing your performance, so the company looks financially stable. That is a tall order because you are attempting to see the future.

It is not easy to achieve the cash objectives and balance your performance. If you need to accumulate $50K for a marketing program, you can simply not pay your rent or vendors, and you will have the money. The problem, of course, is that your balance sheet will not look good (payables will be too high), the landlord may lock you out, and your vendors may not do business with you any longer.

Most poor cash flow management has to do with a lack of planning. You need to know your expected expenses and have an estimate of your sales to do an adequate job of cash flow management. Planning begins with understanding your customer and what drives them to buy from you. Then marketing takes over to get a fresh flow of prospects who qualify to do business with you. Next comes sales to convert those prospects to customers. Then customer service takes the reins to retain the customers for repeat sales or services. All this effort requires cash before you get payment from those customers.

THE MYTH OF PAYING YOURSELF FIRST

When "experts" say to pay yourself first, I am confident they have never been in a bootstrapping business or trying to grow on limited funds. It sounds really lovely to pay yourself first; however, your cash is often tight. If you have $10K in the bank, payroll is $10K, and you need $5K to pay yourself, are you going to pay yourself and allow half of your employees to go unpaid? Unlikely. You will pay them and eke out a little something for yourself. Maybe you should have done a better job of strategizing, raising more money, or any other number of tactics, but faced with reality, you won't pay yourself first! Get real!

CASH FLOW AND THE BUSINESS CYCLE

The business cycle is the cycle of cash into and out of the business:

1. You do work and bill your customer.
2. You put the invoice in accounts receivable.
3. You collect the funds from your customer.
4. You order materials and services from your suppliers.
5. You put their bills in accounts payable.
6. You pay the accounts payable for the expenses of the business.
7. You pay the debts of the business.
8. You make a profit, pay taxes and reinvest in the business.
9. Or you make a profit and take it out of the business for you and your family.
10. The cycle starts again.

Many factors can disrupt this cycle:

1. The customer may not pay or may pay late.
2. Your operating costs may rise.
3. Your staffing may change, causing disruptions in production.
4. Your profits may not be enough to make the necessary investments.
5. You become trapped by the business.

6. Your profits are insufficient to take home the right amount of bacon.

Cash management in the business cycle is about three functions:

1. Plan your business needs: sales, operating expenses, and investments.
2. Do what you need to accelerate the flow of funds into the business.
3. Do what is necessary to slow down the flow of funds out of the business.

If there are only three business cycle functions, why do many companies have problems with cash flow?

- They did a lousy job of planning.
- They did an excellent job planning but ignored the things that could go wrong, like losing a big customer.
- They didn't consider what was needed to invest back in the business.
- They took too much out of the business because "they deserve it; they work so hard."
- They let things happen and didn't manage them.
- They let the inmates run the asylum.
- They did a great job of planning for the short run but didn't plan for the long run.
- They needed to be more strategic in operating the business.

MindSmarts.com has a straightforward cash flow management calculator (CFMS) to help people plan their cash flow. It starts with a budget. In the chapter on pricing, you learned about the planning and High-Performance Brain Training that goes into choosing a price for your product or service. The budget typically includes revenues and expenses. It can consist of planning for bank loans, equipment purchases, and other financings. You are much farther ahead of others in cash flow management when you use a budget. Why?

When you use the CFMS, the first benefit is to have forecasted your cash, so you have an idea of where you stand. A more significant benefit often comes when you ask, "Why? Why did I think my sales would be $X? Why did I think my customers would pay me in 30 days? Why did I think my sales force would produce the sales I needed? Why did I think that I would never lose that big customer? Why did I think my cost of goods was 25%? Why did I underestimate my expenses? Why did I think I could ride my vendors? Why did I think I could get that bank loan? Why did I think my family could live on no cash flow from me?"

With questions based on your original forecast, you will begin to handle the cash flow issues more successfully by innovating strategies to overcome the shortfalls in your plan.

BUSINESS FAILURE AND CASH FLOW

If you have desperate problems with cash flow and a lack of liquidity, you must implement innovation protocols. Most business owners will be operating in panic mode at this point in their careers. Let me assure you that almost everyone survives the worst financial setbacks.

In my case, I bought a company that built bank buildings. With a national change in tax laws, the market for my business disappeared. Investor partners took over the assets of my company;

my wife wanted me to move to take a job, and I had used a lot of my funds to start the business in the first place. But through the brainpower of paradox, I could recognize the mistakes and recover. That is when I formed my accounting practice.

Almost every business failure is preceded by operating losses that suck the liquidity out of the business. At other times the investment of liquid assets into long-term investments (fixed assets like equipment and real estate) sucks up the liquidity so that current liabilities cannot be paid. But that's not the problem. Cash flow problems are the result of issues, not the cause. It really goes back to planning. You must dig even deeper into the problem.

While lack of planning precedes cash flow problems, the planning may be throughout all business areas. Poor planning may relate to sales, operations, overhead, management, or ownership. Poor planning may relate to banking relationships or investors. The SBA states that in 40% of business failures, the owner did not understand the market for their product or service. Wow, that is huge. If you think your service is the best thing since sliced bread and it isn't, all the planning in the world won't solve that problem. Cash flow issues can come from all elements of the cash flow cycle.

Cash flow problems related to sales:

1. The sales don't happen as quickly or in the volume projected.
2. The sales grow too fast in greater volume than projected.
3. The customer pays slower.
4. You have returns or disputes.

Cash flow problems related to purchasing:

1. Quality and cost of your purchases.
2. Deciding whether you need the purchase at all.
3. The timing of when you pay.

When you start with forecasting the easy stuff, for many businesses, this means purchasing. You can rely on the protocol of zooming in to understand the details surrounding the costs and delivery of what you need.

Cash flow problems related to operations, overhead, and ownership:

All areas of the business have the same possible issues and questions relating to cash flow. Do you need to spend the money in the first place? Can you spend it differently? When will you let go of the cash?

A BAD PLAN IS BETTER THAN NO PLAN

Not being strategic and not planning means flying blind. Flying blind means you will get somewhere different than where you intended. Getting somewhere else at an unexpected time means CASH FLOW PROBLEMS. Remember, cash flow is a timing issue.

The reality is that any plan, even one that is wrong, is better than no plan. What? Why is that? It is because you can ask yourself two questions about any planned item:

1. Did the real world look like the plan?
2. Why did I think the plan was realistic in the first place?

Let me give an example. You have a new product, and you have no idea how much you will sell. Plan anyway. "I plan to sell $1,000,000 of this product in the first year beginning in January." You translate this to $83,333 per month for 12 months. The year ends, and you sell $400,000.

It is easy to see you sold $600K less than the plan. The more important part is, "Why did I think I would do $1,000,000 in the first place?"

When you answer this, you will know how to make a better plan for the following year. The answer may involve your available time, hiring a sales rep, marketing costs, etc. You may learn that you are now at $83K a month; it just took time to get started. You may discover a seasonal cycle on your new product that would cause cash flow issues; you can now do a better job of being strategic. Just because you plan for a year, remember that you can jump into the plan in the middle of the year and revise it when you have more information.

JUST BORROW IT

If you have done an excellent job of planning, you may have borrowing capacity, so just borrow it…from a bank or investors. When borrowing from the bank, they want you to have good cash flow so that you can pay them back. When borrowing from an investor, they want the same things as the bank; however, if you don't pay them back they may take over your company so the stakes are much higher.

FINAL THOUGHT

Throughout the process of cash flow management, you can use the High-Performance Brain Training protocols to switch from short-term decision-making to being a strategic thinker. Remember that you are already thinking about your business issues; by thinking about them differently, you will grow your brain's white matter, increase the blood flow, recapture the lost cognitive capital, and make better business decisions. With better brain health and better business decisions, you will be in control of your cash flow instead of it controlling you. Doesn't that sound good?

KEY TAKEAWAYS

- Cash flow issues are often the RESULT of other problems, not the CAUSE.
- The timing of cash creates the most problems for business owners.
- Use strategic attention to tackle tasks that impact cash flow.
- Bootstrapping creates good habits that help a business survive using innovation protocols of High-Performance Brain Training.
- Most poor cash flow management is directly linked to a lack of planning; a bad plan is better than no plan.
- Remember that you are already thinking about your business issues; by thinking about them differently, you will grow your brain's white matter, increase the blood flow, recapture the lost cognitive capital, and make better business decisions. Sounds good, doesn't it?
- Better brain health and better business decisions prevent your cash flow from controlling YOU.

CHAPTER

MARKETING 101

Before starting this chapter, you need to put yourself in the position of your customer. To do this, use the protocols in strategic attention to give you the space to find clarity. Remember that doing two things at once, no matter how popular multi-tasking is, is toxic to your brain. Your brain is not wired to do it. Then identify two elephants that move your needle forward. For example, one elephant may be to gain an understanding of what marketing is; another might be to analyze and choose a particular marketing strategy. Don't forget to take brain breaks throughout this process to let your brain assimilate your new marketing knowledge and incorporate it into your thinking.

Your knowledge of marketing is so important because:

1. The SBA says about 40% of businesses fail because there is no market for their product. If you have customers, ask them why they bought from you. Learn from them. Ask questions.
2. Marketing precedes almost everything in a business. Poor marketing results are described as other problems (cash

flow, client loss, personnel problems) but often go back to the fundamental marketing problem of identifying enough qualifying prospects.

There are only two reasons for marketing:

1. It moves people away from some fear or problem they have.
2. It drives people to something they want (money, power, peace).

Easy isn't it? Not really! It is if you know your customer, yourself, and what you do. If you know your customer, that is a significant starting point. The best customer in the world may not be the best for you. If you are not focused, committed, knowledgeable, trustworthy, and helpful, that customer may not be your best customer for a long time. If you don't understand what you do, you won't be able to justify the two reasons for marketing.

CLARITY

If you think about what I described, it is really about clarity. If you understand your customer, you will know what fears or problems they have, and you will know that your product/service will help them get what they want.

Let's discuss the concept of clarity. If you have clarity, you can speak, advertise, market, write about, or demonstrate how your product/service will move people away from the fear or problem they have or help them get what they want. Let me give you an example. I am a CPA. If I say, "We will do your tax return professionally and timely," that is nothing. What if I say instead, "We will save you money on your taxes and keep the IRS off your doorstep?" This would be better.

From a brain performance standpoint, gaining clarity will give you the focus necessary to attack your roadmap with the proper intention and energy. Typically you will gain clarity by zooming in on the details and zooming out to understand the trends behind your business activities. Zooming deep and wide will allow you to view your ideas as an extension of yourself and how you want your company to be known…your legacy.

GET YOUR MIND RIGHT
CONFUSION AND LACK OF CLARITY = NO TRUST

1. Your relationship with a customer is a trust relationship. They will buy from you because they trust you to deliver.
2. If they get confused, they will not buy from you.
3. If you get confused, you will sell them the wrong thing or the right thing at the wrong time.

When understanding the concept of clarity vs. confusion from a Brain Performance standpoint, it is necessary to use the innovation protocols for a broader understanding. Using the brainpower of infinite, recognize an infinite number of possibilities for your product or service and how it responds to your customer needs. When you are innovative in this way, you will be able to find a way to communicate with clarity so that your customer moves from fear to peace. Your communication will eliminate confusion that can destroy trust.

YOUR IDEAL CLIENT

So, let's start with your customer. Write a story about your best client. Please include all the ways they will interact with you. If they act differently, they will lose trust, or you will lose trust. Let's pick two elements of a customer relationship as examples:

Personality: If you and your company regularly interact with your customer, your ideal client may be joyful, helpful, and understanding. Suppose you have a prospective client with a sour personality, griping, unhappy, ungrateful, etc. In that case, you may not want them as a client (unless you are a psychologist) regardless of everything else. This is a case of the bad apple spoiling the whole barrel.

Problem Solving: Will the client work with you to find a solution for a problem, or will they put it all on you and accept no responsibility for their part? If the problem is you, you need to correct it. If the problem is the client, you may not want to work with them in the future.

Because KepnerCPA is in the service business, we must be able to trust our clients. We have determined that the trust will be broken or minimized if there is any confusion in the relationship. Our clients expect a lot from us. We expect a lot from them. We believe that the way to describe the ideal client is to write a story about them.

In this section, I will walk you through defining your ideal client. First, refer to the Ideal Client Scene for KepnerCPA (**Appendix A**) at the end of this book). Read through it and identify the following traits and characteristics which will help you write your Ideal

Client Scene. Describe your relationship with your client in the following terms:

- Mutual respect
- Personality
- Honesty
- Challenging
- Willingness to accept something new
- Able to recognize benefits
- Your internal benefits
- Trust
- Buys from the company, not one person
- Problem solver
- Pays bills
- Meets commitments
- Thankfulness
- View you as an integral partner
- Will freely promote you and the benefits they have received
- View you as long-term
- Strategic

This Ideal Client exercise will take an investment on your part. I guarantee that you will have a much clearer understanding of your client. From a Brain Performance perspective, beginning to see your client as an extension of your company and your own personal legacy will require zooming deep and wide to see how the client fits. By using these protocols, you are solving a significant need for your company's success and growing the white matter and blood flow in your brain. Remember, your brain loves to be challenged. Defining the ideal client and measuring your other clients against it is a challenging proposition.

"Wait a minute, Kep. I am selling a $50 product. I only want a customer who pays me, one who doesn't return my product, and one with whom I don't have to interact." OK! Write that up. You can gain clarity that to have this type of customer, you have to deliver exactly what you promised when you promised, and of the right quality, so it doesn't get returned. You could also make returns easy, so you don't have to interact with this ideal customer.

WHAT MARKETING STRATEGIES ARE RIGHT FOR YOU?

Only after you know your ideal client can you consider marketing strategies.

1. These clients are ideal. You want more of these prospects, so choose strategies to find more. You can begin to exclude those who are not ideal.
2. We have identified only two reasons they bought from you: 1. To move away from a fear or problem. 2. To drive them to something they want, not need.
3. We have discussed the need for clarity. Without clarity, your message will be lost in your marketing strategy, and you will lose trust.

Many of you reading this book should stop at this point because you have a lot to do to understand your client and gain clarity about what your client wants. High-Performance Brain Training builds focus and clarity. The success of your business at its foundation requires your focus and clarity. Lack of focus has killed far more businesses than lack of capital. Give your brain what it needs.

There are over 40 different strategies you might try for your business. It isn't enough to say you want to market; you must develop a marketing strategy to attract the kind of customer you want. When you consider that you may combine strategies and use several at once, the selection of marketing strategies becomes even more complex. The MindSmarts course on Marketing 101 discusses some of these strategies, but your selection may change from time to time. You may even need a marketing professional or coach to help you choose. Please refer to the 41 marketing strategies (**Appendix B**) at the end of this book.

Marketing is often thought of as lead generation. Lead generation is discussed in "The Funnel" section of this chapter. The challenging part of marketing is what you have already been doing. Defining your ideal client or customer and gaining clarity about them, you, and your product/service is the difficult strategic part of marketing.

THE FUNNEL

You have probably heard of a sales funnel. At the top of the funnel, your advertising or marketing brings prospects into a connection with your company. The initial goal is to remind them of the pain or fears and the joys and desires. Usually, the stronger identity is with pain or fear. Once they are reminded, there are two elements to moving someone down through the funnel. Firstly, they need to have repeated contact. Secondly, they need to learn more about your company at each connection, information that moves them closer to becoming a customer OR excludes them if they are not going to be ideal for you.

Most marketing is designed to give prospects a chance to qualify you. Flip your thinking around. If you know your ideal client, marketing should qualify prospects that meet your Ideal Client Scene. Because you went through the effort in this book to really understand your customer, your marketing should be designed to include and encourage the prospects that might qualify to do business with you.

This is a very powerful position to be in. Don't be afraid to say that you are not for everyone who interfaces with your marketing. If they can't afford you, you can exclude them. If they are not respectful, you can exclude them. If they don't pay their bills, you can exclude them. If they plan to misuse your product, you can exclude them. Please recognize that the non-ideal customer will cost you far more than you get in revenues. They will take up space and effort that should be directed at your ideal customers.

Thinking about your customers qualifying to do business with you requires innovation. As with most innovative thinking, the brainpower of the unknown says that you cannot always know the outcome of your decisions before they are tested in the real world. Remember that the brainpower of paradox encourages resiliency since tremendous gains come from mistakes or errors.

Through the funnel, you may use multiple marketing strategies. Examples include workshops, assessment tools, industry articles supporting your point of view, a free report, a comparison with competition, a book, or almost anything that would direct prospects to become your ideal client. You can offer these contacts online, in person, at a central location, at your office, or over Zoom. You can offer them through other people, yourself, or your staff. You can offer them at various times, in differing formats, for free, or charge for them. The opportunities are endless.

You can find a lot of information on sales funnels by using your best friend, Google. However, you cannot really understand a funnel for lead generation unless you have done the work to know your client, yourself, and your product/service and gained absolute clarity on the essential three things you have been reading about:

1. You must clearly know your ideal client and all the qualities that make them ideal for you.
2. You must have absolute clarity about who you are to flip your approach to where you expect the client to qualify to do business with you.
3. You must clearly understand the pain and pleasure thresholds to move a prospect to become an ideal customer for you.

When you have this clarity, you have eliminated confusion. When there is no confusion, you can build trust with the customer, the trust that is necessary for any relationship to thrive.

YOUR BRAND

Branding is a significant step in your company and its products or services. Why do pharmaceutical companies put so much effort into branding? It isn't just about the name. In naming our Advisory/Brain Performance service, I started with 200 possible names before arriving at our trademark: MindSmarts.

Pharma looks for symptoms, groups them, and names them. With a brand, everyone can talk about what you do. Your employees can all relate to the brand, and you can incorporate it into all aspects of your business. Your production systems will have the brand. Your marketing will have the brand. Your accounting will have the brand. Your delivery will have the brand. Your attorneys will know the brand. Your sales force will center around the brand. Your logistics will carry the brand. Other professionals will know your brand.

The struggle for most small businesses is how to distinguish themselves from others. I am a CPA; can you think of anything more generic? People automatically think about tax returns or financial statements if I introduce myself as a CPA. As a practical matter, these services are commodities that move people away from their fears. If they are commodities, how can someone distinguish themselves? Think H&R Block or KepnerCPA.

The second part of the brand is the one-liner that describes it. The one-liner for KepnerCPA is "Your Prosperity – Our Purpose." Following our core values, we deliver services to our clients that relieve them of the fear of the IRS or of being trapped in their business. Following our core values, we respect our employees and empower them to take responsibility for their knowledge and growth, providing them prosperity.

We have named our advisory services MindSmarts with the one-liner of "Science on the Right Side of Business." This name incorporates our vision of "unlocking business prosperity and owner wealth through brain performance and proven business principles." The one-liner puts the science from the Center for BrainHealth behind the business owner as they make important management decisions.

Branding consolidates all the heavy lifting you have been putting your brain through. Here you have to use all of the Brain Performance protocols to comprehensively analyze and assimilate the full scope of what you do and the clients you serve. You must consider how you want your company to be seen and recognized.

You have to use all the integrated reasoning protocols as you analyze the elements that go into your brand. Using the innovative protocols of Brain Performance, you can overcome similar names, like services and communication issues. You can creatively define your differences and broadcast them to your ideal clients and prospects.

To give you perspective, it took about three months to arrive at the MindSmarts brand even though we have had a consulting platform for years and studied High-Performance Brain Training for three years. Our branding included choosing the name, buying the URL, selecting the graphics, choosing music, and learning how to represent the brain. In addition, it took hundreds of hours to format the material so it could be delivered to business owners like yourself.

YOUR ONE-PAGE MARKETING PLAN

To focus on your marketing plan, I challenge you to put it on one page to achieve the greatest clarity. I learned this lesson years ago when raising money for a business. The financing was agreed to in 5 minutes with an investment banker named Bob Welborn. The entire business plan was 100+ pages that I had to explain in that 5 minutes. I could do that only by having a one-page business plan to give me clarity. Your plan should include the following:

- Executive summary - your brand and your mission
- Describe your target market
- Competitors?
- Economic, environmental, political, cultural, and regulatory forces
- Impact of technology

- What distinguishes you from competitors
- Benefits to your clients and you
- Current marketing performance
- Financial targets and staffing
- Financial summary
- What is next?

KEY TAKEAWAYS

- Marketing precedes almost every other aspect of a business.
- Marketing moves people away from fears or problems and drives them towards things they want (money, power, peace).
- It is imperative to have clarity when developing your marketing message.
- Define your ideal client and prioritize trust in the relationship.
- Select marketing strategies that will attract your ideal client.
- Use sales funnels to lure in ideal clients OR exclude ones who will not meet your ideal client criteria.
- Brand effectively by analyzing and assimilating the full scope of what you do and the clients you serve using Brain Performance protocols. You must consider how you want your company to be seen and recognized.

CHAPTER

FINANCING YOUR BUSINESS

As a practical matter, everyone needs financing at times in their business lives. One of the major mistakes is borrowing long-term money for short-term needs. A worse mistake is borrowing short-term money for long-term needs. Let's dig into this further. Both methods tie up your funds, leaving you trapped for the short run. In this chapter, I will introduce you to a wonderful tool for any business; you may have seen the Ansoff Matrix before. As you see it used in this book, apply it to other business issues you are facing. Examine the Ansoff Matrix below to match funds with uses. You can apply this matrix to any number of business decisions, including matching short and long-term funds with uses.

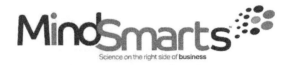

	Short Term	Long Term
Source of Funds	• Credit Cards • Lines of Credit • Sales & A/R	• Bank • Mortgage • Equipment Leases • Investment
Use of Funds	• Expenses • Advertising • Lender A/P • Office	• Building Equipment

When looking at the short-term versus the long-term needs and funding sources, you will use all brain protocols to understand this issue. You will use zooming in to understand the need for the funds fully. You will use zooming out to think about themes and understand the sources of funds and whether short-term or long-term. Zooming deep and wide will help you know the goal for the funding and the investment of the dollars as it affects the business and your personal life. Zooming deep and wide, you will challenge your willingness to grow your business.

Using the brainpower of infinite, you will understand the wide variety of funding sources and the effect they may have on your banking and other lenders. Using the brainpower of paradox, you will be alert to how the matching of uses and sources is going and be willing to adjust your plans if things are not going just right. The brainpower of the unknown will allow you to match sources with uses; even if they don't match fully, you will have broadened your knowledge and created a stronger foundation for the future. You must become resilient when it comes to borrowing funds.

FINANCING IS REQUIRED FOR MOST BUSINESSES

The cash flow chapter in this book shows why almost every business needs to borrow. The cash from sales does not come into the business as fast as the expenses go out. You must have the borrowing capacity to cover the gap. It is more than just having enough cash to pay your bills. If you don't have enough to invest in your business, you may need to borrow or be trapped in your business.

We learned about being strategic to solve your cash needs. The old joke is that you don't need to borrow until you don't qualify. It may be a joke, except when the joke is on you. Good planning allows you to develop banking relationships with lines of credit before you need them. Good planning inspires confidence from a lender. Good planning inspires confidence in you. Don't expect to get suitable financing from your banker next Friday for payroll; they may ask why you waited until now. Don't you think it makes sense to transform your thinking into a strategy and put some financing in place before you need it?

Let's use the Ansoff Matrix again on "strategic versus no strategy" and "having resources versus having no resources." The correct strategy depends on the quadrant that your company falls in.

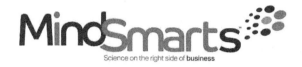

	Save	Invest
Strategic		
No Strategy	Spend	Squander
	No Resources	Resources

A tool like the Ansoff matrix focuses your brain and allows you to create an innovative solution. Using a tool like this means you don't have to think about how to solve the problem in the short term. You can be strategic in your problem-solving. Being strategic is like a double boost to the brain. You are being innovative in how you face the problem and being strategic and solving the issue at hand. Don't forget that your brain's white matter actually grows; it is the transportation highway between your frontal lobe and the amygdala, the center for memory and emotion. That seems like a good thing to me!

USING TOMORROW'S MONEY FOR TODAY

Most borrowing is using tomorrow's money today or covering up for the cash spent for past uses. Do you need money today? Google "I need money today" or "My business needs money today." This may take you to www.nerdwallet.com, and you can get immediate funds. Isn't this great?! You can get the money almost immediately to get your business over the cash crunch. You can make payroll after all or make your house payment. You can breathe again. Or can you? You just hit your credit score with a high-cost loan, revealing to everyone you are in trouble. You made it more difficult to borrow at better terms because of the cost of today's loan.

Please don't do this unless you promise never to do it again. Having money is like a drug. You need it; you want it; you can get it; you don't have to deal with your real problems. Needing expensive short-term money is like a gambler's fix. Why? Because the owner bets that sales and profits will come in fast enough to cover their bet (their loan) and the interest cost. They also bet they can overcome the ding on their credit from having to borrow high-cost short-term money.

Remember that hoping is a poor strategy. When you think differently about the things that matter to you, you grow your cognitive reserves. Solving problems is the kind of work your frontal lobe likes; analyzing, cataloging, planning, strategizing, and comparing. Don't confuse action with strategy.

FINANCING FROM YOUR CUSTOMERS OR VENDORS

When looking for financing, look no further than your own customers and vendors. Think about all the money that comes through your business. Most of the dollars in and out are from your customers and vendors. When you think of customers, think about how you can get more money sooner and keep it longer. When you think of vendors, consider how you can spend less money and delay paying them.

Your Customers

You can give volume purchase discounts to increase the overall money, particularly when the added volume allows you to cut your costs. At MindSmarts.com, it is possible to pre-order courses that are not completed yet; can you do this? We have a client that sells software upgrades to some of their larger customers as custom work. My clients end up with programmed features now available in their standard product. The large clients funded the entire increase in new features that my client sells to others without incurring added costs.

Create a loyalty award for your customers; it costs very little and moves them to give you long-term revenue. You get financing when you have a profitable subscription method if you don't have to do extra work to deliver on your promises.

Birds of a feather do flock together. If you encourage your ideal customers to refer others to you, those referrals will likely be the same kind of clients. Look at this as financing your marketing costs.

What is the brain tip behind customer financing? Zoom in to measure your costs for production, delivery, and sales, so you know your costs. Zoom out to understand the themes about how customers react to you as a vendor, including what responsibilities they take on saving you time and money. Zoom deep and wide to understand how you want your company to be perceived, including your wide range of independent, self-reliant customers. What a great legacy for your business to gain profits because you understood your customers and trained them to be the kind of customers you wanted.

Your Vendors

Every time a vendor sells you on credit, they provide financing. You can ask for volume discounts or payment terms such as 2/10 net 30. 2/10 net 30 is designed to give customers a discount of 2% to pay now, but they have to pay in a month. That sounds cheap, but the 2% is only for ten days; that converts to an interest rate of 36.7% compared to your bank rate of 6% to 8%. You should not give it to your customers, but you should try to get it from your vendors.

Almost everything you do has credit attached to it. The employee who works for you and gets paid on payday has been extending you credit until they get paid. When you use this broad definition of credit, you can see an opportunity to receive credit on almost any cost you incur to fund your company.

If you can extract longer payment terms from a vendor, that means better financing. Several years ago, Texas Instruments notified all their vendors that they would pay bills in 45 days, not 30 days. If a vendor wanted to sell to TI, they had to accept the new terms. Just this 15-day adjustment to vendor payables gave TI $100,000,000 in credit. Like your customers, you can offer a "Vendor of the Year" trophy to keep your costs down. That $145 trophy is worth getting a 10% discount on a million dollars worth of materials.

How else can you get financing from a vendor? You can be a guinea pig for new products to secure a better price. You can allow a vendor to put materials in your unused warehouse space and pay for it only when you need it. Your supplier can become your R&D department by developing special products or services for you. You can even form joint ventures with them to get more from your dollar.

You can ask a vendor to train your sales staff or develop a financing program for your customers.

FINANCING PROVIDED BY YOUR BANKER

Your banker will be your friend if you make it easy for them to loan to you and adhere to the terms of the deal. Bankers have bosses too. The Federal Reserve has a complex funding system to ensure banks remain solvent. The Federal Reserve system is beyond the scope of this lesson; however, someone has to keep an eye on banks so that they can fulfill their obligations to the Fed and their customers.

Assuming the credit risk of loaning to you and other businesses requires that the borrowers meet their end of the bargain by meeting the terms of the borrowing agreement. Here is what happens:

1. You go to your friendly banker. You tell him what you want. He wants to loan you money.
2. Your friendly banker asks you to provide all sorts of information, including financial statements, tax returns, a business plan, a personal financial statement, etc. If you don't have this information, your request might be dead in the water already.
3. Your friendly banker gives all this information to the not-so-friendly credit analyst in the back room for review.
4. The credit analyst looks at your request and documents and assesses whether you can repay the loan.
5. The credit analyst also pulls your credit report. Those late pays, etc., pop up. The credit analyst also calculates the amount of debt you have compared to your company's performance. They report back to your friendly banker.

6. Your friendly banker (remember he wants to loan you money) says the bank would like to do business with you, but you have to provide some other answers. Why is your company losing money? Why is your credit score what it is? What was this bankruptcy eight years ago? What is this lawsuit you are facing? Assuming you satisfy the friendly banker, he will take it to the committee.
7. You hope your friendly banker is a good salesperson. They have to sell the loan committee on why they should loan to you.
8. If the loan committee turns you down, you may have to go to another bank or provide more assurances for this bank.
9. You say that you will guarantee the loan. So what? You would have to do that anyway.
10. If the loan committee agrees with the loan, along comes another set of paperwork with all the reporting requirements. You better be sure your books are up to date.
11. If the loan committee says they will do the loan as an SBA loan, that means more time and paperwork before you get the money. Let me interject. An SBA loan is not a loan from the Small Business Administration. The SBA guarantees 70% of the bank's loan to you. Whoops! More pressure on the bank; if you don't make good on the loan and others are in the same boat, the bank could lose its ability to get SBA guarantees.
12. You hope that you estimated correctly and only need what you asked for. Nothing is worse than going back to the bank and asking for more money, especially if you haven't proven that you can perform on the first loan.

Banks can offer various loans, including lines of credit, high-limit credit cards, term loans, mortgage loans, and a comprehensive combination of terms and amounts in multiple formats. They will try to match the terms of the loans against the collateral; a five-year note for a truck purchase, an eight-year note for plant equipment, and a line of credit for operating costs. Get acquainted with a local banker.

One of the types of loans a bank may offer is an SBA loan, mainly if you are considered a higher risk for your bank. SBA refers to the Small Business Administration. This federal agency doesn't loan money (the exception has been in this COVID world); it guarantees loans made by banks. Because your loan needs a guarantee, you can expect some higher costs and more paperwork, but you are more likely to get the loan.

If you are using the integrated reasoning protocols to negotiate with your banker, start by learning about banks in general. Evaluate the possibility that the bank may be too big for you. It may be convenient, but you are just a number. Evaluate whether the friendly banker has been with the bank for a while and is in a position to help you. Determine what the bank needs by asking the friendly banker what your financial statements must show to get a loan. Know the answer before you ask for the money.

FINANCING PROVIDED BY YOUR FAMILY AND FRIENDS

I started my business using my credit cards and savings. What a pain, but it worked. I used an SBA loan to buy another CPA practice. I used my own resources to start and build my practice. That is the way most people start. And I was like many of those startups; I got behind on credit card payments and had issues but worked out of them.

I am so glad my kids, Aunt Bessie, and my friends are not partners in my business. The holiday dinners would have been ruined if I had been performing poorly. The holiday dinners would have been ruined if I was performing well, and they wanted more income from their loans to me. My friends might not be my friends anymore.

CROWDSOURCING AND KICKSTARTING

A better opportunity can be a kickstarter campaign. Visit www.kickstarter.com to find examples of how people have raised money for their businesses from strangers. Other options include a variety of crowdsourcing opportunities. There are many of these options available today. People are looking for investment opportunities. Crowdfunding is a source of these opportunities. There are new opportunities every day. You can look at MicroVentures, AngelList, Yieldstreet, SeedInvest, Crowdcube, Wefunder, Funding Circle, Companisto, and many others.

Here is how it works. You put your idea out in the crowdsourcing marketplace with a proposal. Let's say you need $50K to complete the design of your product. You plan to manufacture a product for $20 and sell it for $100. For a $50 investment in your company, the investor will get the product for $50. You get your $50K, a boatload of customers (paying a discounted price) to talk about your product and find out if there is demand for what you sell.

There are some key factors in this approach:

1. These are not real sales to regular customers.

2. You may get bad reviews for your work, so unhappy investors/customers are a double whammy on your product.
3. If it costs you more than the discounted price, you have to cover that overage; you may want your CPA to examine your cost.
4. Even if everything works the way you want, you still haven't identified the best marketing.

KEEP AN OPEN MIND

Almost any company you make a substantial purchase from will offer some type of financing. If you need to buy equipment or services, your supplier will offer to lease them or give you terms for purchase. Should you accept their terms?

Although bank loans are typically the lowest-cost loans, almost anyone can provide financing. At times the terms are better. Be open to who may provide your financing. You can email MindSmarts.com for a white paper entitled "58 Sources of Financing" for some other ideas.

KEY TAKEAWAYS

- One of the major financing mistakes is borrowing long-term money for short-term needs. A worse mistake is borrowing short-term money for long-term needs.
- Financing is required for most businesses because cash doesn't come in as quickly as expenses go out.
- Avoid using tomorrow's money today if you can, or at least know the cost to do so.

- When you think of customers, think about how you can get more money sooner and keep it longer. When you think of vendors, consider how you can spend less money and delay paying them.
- If you are using the integrated reasoning protocols to negotiate with your banker, start by learning about banks in general.
- Financing through friends and family seems easy but can lead to less-than-pleasant family gatherings.
- Use crowdsourcing and kickstarting techniques to raise money for your business through strangers.
- Keep an open mind in terms of the various options for financing.

CHAPTER 10

WHAT KEEPS YOU UP AT NIGHT?

This chapter differs from the previous chapters about pricing, cash flow, marketing, and financing. We will identify a list of possible business problems and demonstrate how High-Performance Brain Training can apply to any business problem.

First, the problems or worries:

1. I need cash now.
2. I am losing my biggest customer (or they are upset).
3. I am losing my most crucial employee.
4. I don't have enough resources to complete the work I have now.
5. I don't have enough time to do everything I need (I am tired).
6. There is no business in the pipeline.
7. My spouse wants me to get a job (this happened to me).
8. I am working hard and not earning enough.
9. I can't save for retirement.
10. How can I gain market share without pricing too low?
11. How can I grow my business without losing my special sauce?

12. I have too many people.
13. I have too much business.
14. Who do I hire first?
15. What should my marketing budget be at my stage of business?
16. How can I be innovative in a profitable way?
17. My problem is _____.

You cannot solve all these problems at once. If you solve one of them, how do you know it is the right one to tackle first? What approach should you take to identify and solve the most important problem? You will generally use the same process in tackling any of these problems. You have learned in this book a wide variety of information to use your brain as your best business weapon. So USE IT.

Firstly, you have learned something about brain health and the High-Performance Brain Training protocols that will help get you to the heart of a business problem and solutions that are complete and innovative.

Secondly, you have learned the importance of developing a roadmap and why this differs from goals. Remember that Yogi Berra, the manager of the New York Yankees, said, "If you don't know where you are going, you are going to end up somewhere else."

Finally, this concept has been applied to several business problems, including pricing, cash flow, marketing, and finance. Now it is time to use the protocols to solve the issues that vex you and keep you trapped in an underperforming business. It is estimated that 60% of all small businesses are underperforming; that being the case, the owner is trapped by that business and may not recognize their state.

Because you are operating your business, you can't just stop doing what you are doing and be scholarly to develop what you need in a planned format. If you could do this, you would first define your ideal client, build marketing to attract them, and create your roadmap. While serving your ideal clients, you would build the structural capital to manage the production and deliver on your promise. You probably don't have that luxury, so concentrate on being strategic and long-term in your solutions to any problems you solve. This will minimize the chance that you will have to solve the same problem repeatedly. Identify the problem you want to solve. It may be on the list above or something specific for your business.

USING STRATEGIC ATTENTION

Set aside some time and space to work on the problem. Eliminate distractions and commit to doing only this work (**brainpower of one**). Break down the problem into manageable pieces (**elephants**) using the **brainpower of two**. Remember that elephants require you to use your frontal lobe for categorizing, analyzing, measuring, comparing, and planning; actions that are difficult and require high-level thinking. Solving most problems requires understanding the problem; that can be an elephant in itself. For example, let's say you are being held hostage by a large client.

Your elephants may include:

1. Understanding the magnitude of that significant client individually compared to the company as a whole. They may be the biggest, but that is only 10% of your overall business.
2. Evaluate what you do for them. 10% of your sales is a big deal but not so big if they suck up more than 10% of your resources.

3. The client may be a problem because you use them for training your staff in certain kinds of work.
4. The client may be a lesser problem because the work you do is outdated, and it may not be required in a year anyway.
5. You may have an irrational fear of the effect of the loss on the company.
6. You may be losing the client because they will work only with you, the owner, and not the company.
7. The client may owe you money or pay you consistently so you can count on their funds.

Just defining the problem may be too much for a single elephant. You may have one elephant just to research the client's payment history. Remember to take a brain break of 5 minutes 5 times a day. Brain breaks don't involve "no thought" but are "no effort," allowing your brain to rest and work for you. Think about a brain break as a 5-minute sabbatical from work.

USING INTEGRATED REASONING

If you examine the questions to ask to understand the scope of the problem, you will see the integrated reasoning protocols in use. To understand the facts about any problem, zoom in on the details. This has to do with the characteristics of the work. For example, it could be a client who is 10% of your revenues but using 20% of your resources. When you zoom in, you also know how else the customer interacts with your company.

When you zoom out, you are looking for themes that will impact your understanding of the problem and the possible solutions.

In the case of the large customer holding you hostage, your themes may point out that what is going on with this client is going on with all your clients. It may include the wide range of services you provide to any client, the quality control processes to provide consistency, how you want to structure your company's resources, how you deliver your services, and what is the largest client you ever want to have. These themes are service, QC, setting client expectations, impact on business, leadership, competition, staff compensation, uniqueness of what you offer, brand, and others.

When you zoom deep and wide, you are making this elephant problem and possible solutions personal to you. You may think it is personal simply because of the potential negative financial consequences. However, ask yourself how your company will be perceived by the business community and the other people you interface with. Do you want to be thought of as a company running scared because the business is controlling you or the other way around? Do you personally want to be known as a business owner who is not in charge of your business? Do you want to be the business owner you say you are to your colleagues or the business owner that you know yourself to be…the owner that others do not see? It is exhausting to be one thing to the outside world and another thing to yourself. Zooming deep and wide on a business problem allows you to bring these two pictures of yourself together and make your business reflect how you want to be remembered; your legacy.

INNOVATION

Remember, innovation is the continuous pursuit of original thinking to build new value/meaning/knowledge and shape the future. Once you clearly define the problem you want to solve, you can apply various innovation strategies to find a strategic solution. In fact, even in trying to find the definition of the problem, you will employ some of the brainpower of innovation strategies.

In either problem definition or problem solution, remember that the **brainpower of infinite** tells you there are infinite possibilities. In defining the problem, you only know what you know, so your problem definition may be incomplete; if you broaden your analysis to recognize the infinite nature of things, you will set the foundation for a more innovative solution.

Let me give you an example using the client holding you hostage. In defining the problem, you may identify the truth of the unhappiness, in this case, slow delivery. Your innovative solution may go all the way back to how you communicate with a customer at the front end or explore an infinite number of solutions that will not only solve the problem for this customer but for all of them.

Recognizing that you can't see the future (**brainpower of the unknown**), you don't know how things will work out. But you can strategize the implementation of a solution so you can measure the results as you go along, starting with the large client, so they know you are working on the problem.

You may not need to be reminded that the best results and the most outstanding innovations come from mistakes (**brainpower of paradox**). The problem caused by your large client may be the very best thing for you and your company.

Remember also what you need to succeed:

1. The best use of your greatest business weapon, your brain.
2. Objectivity to view the full scope of your business and its opportunities.

3. Processes on how to tackle your business issues.
4. Trust in yourself or a respected advisor.

We have given you the foundation in this book. You have learned the protocols of High-Performance Brain Training. Some of our clients take this knowledge, ask for added training, and run with it using a DIY (Do It Yourself) model. Some of our clients use us broadly throughout their business to provide objective, independent thinking about their problems. Others seek our assistance to develop their structural capital and culture to grow the value of their business. Finally, some use us to coach them through a single problem or area of their business. If we can help, please let us know. You can reach us at info@MindSmarts.com.

CHAPTER 11

USING HIGH BRAIN PERFORMANCE ON PERSONAL MATTERS

As you know, MindSmarts is about helping someone become a better business owner with more powerful decisions, a sense of optimism and control over their business, and being active in completing the things that are important to them. While using your brain in specific ways, you will not only experience better results, but you will be growing your brain at the same time.

With the power of High-Performance Brain Training, consider using these protocols in other personal ways. If you are not a business owner, you are making a living somewhere. As an employee or manager, you can improve your stature in your company by making better decisions in your role. Wherever there are people, there can be conflict. Using the High-Performance Brain Training, you will be more effective as a manager and employee in resolving those conflicts.

Put yourself in the position of the company that you work for. In theory, they will promote someone who makes the best business decisions and accomplishes the most. That is a broad generalization, but whatever you face will be handled with a higher component of knowledge and grace as you meet and achieve your employer's expectations. Of course, you will also face some limitations, for example, the boss that demands you complete the wrong things to stroke their ego. But think about it! If you use all the protocols in this book, you will come up with better solutions for your career, even if it means you seek other employment.

Remember the brainpower of two: two elephants daily that you can complete in 45 minutes each that move your needle forward either personally or professionally. An example might be to take the High-Performance Brain Training at MindSmarts.com and break it into a dozen elephants so you can integrate these powerful protocols into your daily life. After completing that work, you may define an elephant to discover how to become a Brain Healthy Workplace for your department or entire company. Using the protocols makes you the ideal candidate to promote this training company-wide.

Another very personal area to consider for needing better analysis and brain training is your family. I hope I haven't opened Pandora's box. Just look around; many families have problems that require a fresh approach. Unfortunately, we all get stuck in a particular approach to a family problem because our emotions are stronger than in other arenas we operate in. Let's examine a case study and see how to apply High-Performance Brain Training.

John and Mary have two children. They are estranged from Mary's cousin, Alice. Alice used to be connected to the family and attend family functions but has not done so for several years. As I have said, I am not a brain scientist. I am also not a psychologist. If I were, I would include many other details about the family dynamics that are not present here. The idea is for you to "fill in the blanks" for a family situation you are facing.

With all the history and the emotion attached, your fresh approach using the Brain Training protocols can't be implemented during or immediately after family interaction when the emotions are raw. Instead, start with the strategies related to STRATEGIC ATTENTION.

1. **The Brainpower of One:** Set aside time when you will not be interrupted. Remember that your brain is not wired to do two things at once. A business owner would shut their door or tell his admin to hold his calls or sit in the conference room or a vacant office (or even go offsite) to limit distractions.

2. **The Brainpower of Two:** Define two elephants relating to the family dynamic that can be completed in 45 minutes each. Why 45 minutes? That's as long as the brain can concentrate on an issue without becoming unfocused. Let's consider what those elephants may look like:

You will not be able to have an elephant described as "Determine why the relationship with Alice is the way it is and come up with a dynamic solution to change that relationship." That is way too big an expectation, so break it down.

A series of elephants may each examine the lives of the estranged family members. Instead of being **person-based**, they might be broken up into **age-based** analysis. How did the families interact as children, teens, or adults? They might be **event-based**, remembering some events that affected the relationships.

1. **Take Brain Breaks:** You may spend time on an Alice elephant (or a John elephant or a Mary "as a teen" elephant), but you may not experience any "aha "moments during your work. Your brain needs to rest to work for you. I always have my "aha" moments in the mornings after I have rested. Writing this chapter is an example of how my brain rested last night and guided me to complete the writing this morning.

The manner in which you work on your elephants is where the INTEGRATED REASONING protocols come into play. You have set your time to attack your issues; now, use all the power of INTEGRATED REASONING to bear on the problems. Remember that your brain thrives on handling complex problems. Your brain's white matter grows. Your blood flow increases. The neurons in your frontal lobe become more connected and powerful. Your frontal lobe is where your executive function operates to evaluate, plan, assess, measure, decide, prioritize, analyze, and strategize all parts of your handling of this important family matter.

1. **Power of Zooming In:** Zooming in is where you get the details. With a family matter, you often have to look at more than just the current players. Remember that the apple doesn't fall too far from the tree. People may comment on the physical resemblance in a family, but the same can be said for the emotional and relationship dynamics. I have always been clear that I am not my Dad, but when I am being insightful, I see characteristics of his that I embody. As you work on your chosen elephant, zoom in to the powerful forces that make each person who they are.

2. **Power of Zooming Out:** Zooming out is about analyzing in "themes." Themes could be witnessed in how Alice interacts with males in the family differently than females. Themes might exist from childhood that relate to actions as someone tries to gain independence from their parents. Themes make you see situations from a much broader perspective. For example, understanding the pattern of substance abuse would change someone's understanding of a problem and identify different solutions.
3. **Power of Zooming Deep and Wide:** Using the power of zooming deep and wide is a way to make the situation personal to you. But this is family; it is already personal. While you may be involved with the situation, understanding how the problem and solution will affect you personally will make it more meaningful. Let's say you are Bill, and Alice is in Mary's family. You may care about the impact on Mary and others in the family, but when you examine it from your personal perspective, you will have a stronger connection to the Alice issue. Zooming deep and wide is about creating new meaning and applying it to personal contexts by combining your knowledge and experience.

In the business owner's case, I think of zooming deep and wide as a legacy issue; how do you want to be remembered as a business owner? Take it to the family level. What do you want your legacy to be; involved, caring, solver of family problems, abdicating your relationship? Zooming deep and wide will make it personal and get you where you want to be remembered.

As you analyze the family situation, you will probably have to be innovative. Using the High-Performance Brain Training protocols for INNOVATION will help you find innovative solutions for your family issue. Think about it; as you have dealt with the problem in the past, you may have begun limiting the possible solutions for the family issue. We all have a habit of limiting our possible solutions because "We tried that, and it didn't work," "She won't agree to that," "That will ruin Christmas,"...the list of reasons goes on.

Remember the definition of INNOVATION as you apply it to your family. INNOVATION is the continuous pursuit of original thinking to build new value/meaning/knowledge and shape the future.

Perhaps you will conclude that the problem won't be solved. That may be the outcome, and then part of the innovation will be to accept this in the best possible way. Or it may be to wait until some trigger event changes the dynamics (a marriage, a college graduation, an illness, etc.).

Perhaps your solution is strengthening good relationships, thus keeping the doors open for later reconciliation. Maybe it is as simple as apologizing for something.

1. **The Brainpower of Infinite:** This protocol is to recognize that there are an infinite number of possible solutions. Each person in the family has a unique relationship with the other members. For a family of 10, there are 45 individual relationships, not to mention groups such as Bill and Mary, with the other eight family members. Just think what this means as you attempt to find a solution for the Alice issue.

It is not enough to just think about the relationships within the family. What if Mary belongs to a social group and one other person in the family belongs as well? Then what if that family member belongs to another group that Alice is a member of? Perhaps it is not a social group; it is an employer. Identifying these relationships may not mean anything, but it gives you more information as you analyze the issue and possible solutions.

1. **The Brainpower of Paradox:** This protocol is about your resilience. Throughout your life, you have tried things like riding a bicycle. You didn't know the thrill or the consequences until you fell by jumping the curb. You can apply this to your family mystery. Maybe it isn't Alice, but Mary had a childhood experience that caused her to be wary of some behavior exhibited by Alice. If Mary hasn't developed resilience about this issue, the Alice issue will continue to be a problem.

We may not like to make errors or mistakes; I don't know anyone who likes to do that. However, a mistake is the greatest opportunity for growth. I have made a lot of mistakes in my life, and I hope I never stop making mistakes. I have learned that I can recover from any mistake; it may be painful and take a long time, but I will recover. Trying innovative actions in your family may prove that you will recover as well.

1. **The Brainpower of the Unknown:** When you are innovative, you can analyze, strategize, and plan all you want, but you cannot know the outcome before it happens. Let's take Alice; you choose an innovative solution of getting the cousins together to integrate Alice into the family, only to push her further away. Instead, you choose an innovative solution

of not inviting her to a family get-together, hoping she will miss it; that pushes her away. So, two opposite strategies; you can only know the result once you implement them.

This protocol is about cultivating curiosity and opening yourself up to being a change creator, not a change blocker. Mark Cuban, NBA owner, and Shark Tank investor, recently mentioned "seeking curiosity" as necessary for an entrepreneur, so it is for all business owners. Do you think you already know your family and all of its dynamics? Just think of when one of your kids (now an adult) told you something they did, and you had no clue. At the business level, cultivating curiosity is about implementing change in your business. At the family level, it is about caring about the people nearest to you.

Make your life as a business owner, a family member, a friend, a mentor, a participator, a student, or a person the most meaningful life it can be. Invest in yourself with MindSmarts.

Learn more about MindSmarts High-Performance Brain Training and our workshops at **www.MindSmarts.com**

OR

Are you interested in High-Performance Brain Training or coaching? Your first Discovery session is **FREE**. Email **info@MindSmarts.com** or call Kep personally at **214-361-5081**

APPENDIX

A

THE IDEAL CLIENT SCENE FOR KEPNER CPA

Our ideal client values our work and counsel. They want to learn and grow their business. They will listen to us and want us to teach them about financial and business matters. They will view us as their key advisor when they deal with other professionals, such as attorneys, financial planners, etc. They will have a sense of humor and see us as an integral part of their business, not as a vendor. They will be honest in their dealings with other parties and with us, and with their employees and customers.

Our ideal client knows what they are buying and when their requests require extra work. The work we do for them will be challenging and interesting, allowing us to expand our staff with experienced, skilled professionals such as CPAs and CEPAs. All professionals from our firm that work with the client will learn something and will be able to grow in knowledge, experience, and skill from what they learn. What we learn from one of these clients can be applied to other clients.

They will embrace MindSmarts Brain Performance protocols and use the tools to enhance their own learning and skills. They will integrate these protocols into their daily lives and have an increase in all areas of their lives as an overall benefit of their use.

We will be able to document our projects for these clients and develop programs and systems that can be used as templates for work for other clients. We can manage these developed programs so that other staff can implement them for different clients, and Kep's time will be only for the most extensive and creative opportunities.

Our ideal client will trust that we will work hard on their behalf and give them professional and helpful results. They will not expect Kep to do their work but expect him to supervise it. They will work well with our staff and develop a relationship with them. They will be so happy with the work we prepare for them and our relationship with them that they will refer other similar clients to us.

If there is a problem, they will work with us to resolve it and not view it as a "them vs. us" issue. We will be part of the solution, not part of the problem. In return, we will handle all matters promptly and efficiently for them and give them abundant exchanges, including matters with outside agencies and internal issues in either their office or ours. If there is a problem, they will come to us and work with us to resolve it. They will be patient with us, and we will be with them.

They will pay us well and receive benefits well in excess of our fees. They will implement business strategies that will give them substantial growth in the value of their business. They will recognize the value of our work and will happily provide referrals to others about the work we have done and the benefits they have received.

As they grow, they will not replace us with internal personnel but will see us as value-added support even if they hire an internal CPA with knowledge and experience. They will use us for other meaningful, challenging opportunities to support their company when they grow.

The work for our ideal client will continue for many years in a mutually beneficial and abundant manner.

APPENDIX B

41 MARKETING STRATEGIES

1. Alliance marketing (WHAT)
2. Affiliate marketing (WHAT)
3. Affinity marketing (WHAT)
4. Ambush marketing (HOW)
5. Article marketing (HOW)
6. Brand lover marketing (HOW)
7. B2B marketing (WHAT)
8. B2C marketing (WHAT)
9. Call to action marketing (HOW)
10. Cause marketing (WHAT)
11. Close range marketing (HOW)
12. Cloud marketing (HOW)
13. Community marketing (WHAT)
14. Cross-media marketing (HOW)
15. Cultural marketing (WHAT)
16. Database marketing (HOW)
17. Direct mail marketing (HOW)

18. Diversity marketing (WHAT)
19. Drip marketing (HOW)
20. Email marketing (HOW)
21. Evangelism marketing (WHAT)
22. Event marketing (WHAT)
23. Freebie marketing (HOW)
24. Free sample marketing (HOW)
25. Guerrilla marketing (HOW)
26. Humanistic marketing (WHAT)
27. Inbound marketing (HOW)
28. Link exchanges (HOW)
29. Mass marketing (HOW)
30. Mobile marketing (HOW)
31. Newsletter marketing (HOW)
32. Niche marketing (WHAT)
33. Offline marketing (HOW)
34. Online marketing (HOW)
35. Outbound marketing (HOW)
36. Personalized marketing (WHAT)
37. Promotional marketing (HOW)
38. PR Marketing (HOW)
39. Refer a friend (WHAT)
40. Relationship marketing (WHAT)
41. Reverse marketing (HOW)

ABOUT KEP KEPNER, CPA, CEPA

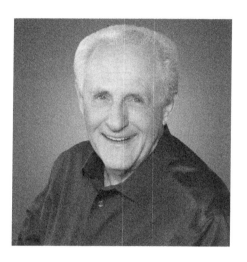

Kep is the founder and namesake managing partner of KepnerCPA and the founder of MindSmarts.com. He came into the accounting profession in an unusual way with a background in sales and marketing from his stint at IBM and other computer companies. His marketing background allowed him to become the partner in charge of the management consulting practice of Alford Meroney & Company, a regional CPA firm. When Alford Meroney merged, Kep became a Management Consulting Partner at Arthur Young.

Kep has an accounting degree from "can't wait until basketball season" Kansas University (Rock Chalk Jayhawk) and an MBA in finance from the University of California – Berkeley. But his education wasn't complete until he cashed in his corner office at Arthur Young to acquire a company that built bank buildings. When that business tanked in the financial debacle of the 1980s (Kep calls that a learning experience), he started KepnerCPA in his spare bedroom.

Through his own experiences and those of his many clients, Kep has identified the factors that separate highly successful companies from also-rans. He has defined those strategic factors in two books and regularly consults with his clients to help them grow and prosper.

No, he doesn't read the tax code every night but deals with it daily. He knows that the best tax strategy is to make money, a lot of it. For a business owner to become prosperous, they have to think differently. A thought precedes every action, so learning to use your brain to think differently and more wisely will result in better decisions and growth in prosperity and wealth for business owners who use MindSmarts.

Kep is more content climbing Aconcagua and Kilimanjaro, swimming in the Arctic Ocean, or taking a horseback trek in outer Mongolia…not the typical life of a CPA. He is happily married to Kim and has two adult sons, Peter and Kyle, who have survived his entrepreneurial efforts without too many scars.

WEBSITE: www.MindSmarts.com
EMAIL: info@MindSmarts.com
PHONE: 214-361-5081

WHAT KEP'S CLIENTS ARE SAYING...

Prior to having Kep work with us using his MindSmarts program, I had a mess on my hands and just couldn't get my business issues managed. We had a $50,000,000 company but were operating out of control. Kep helped me develop a roadmap that put my company on track to operate more efficiently and profitably. His High-Performance Brain Training changed my way of dealing with the problems and cleared the deck for substantial growth in the value of my company.

We have followed the MindSmarts brain training protocols and anticipate further growth now that I feel that our company is under control. Since we are now operating at a higher standard, I am excited about what this year will bring. I recommend that you take the brain training and also hire KepnerCPA to develop your roadmap and help you define and reach your targets.

—Jerry Powell
LSPM, LLC

While I have a successful business, the COVID world, and the pressure in our industry to be environmentally friendly, I am always faced with business decisions and want to make the best decisions possible. I took the MindSmarts High-Performance Brain Training in a workshop offered by KepnerCPA and have embraced the technology. Like everything else worthwhile, you have to have some diligence to get the most out of it, but its concepts are simple and easy to use.

To prove the importance, I took my two daughters to meet with Kep to let them gain some understanding about the innovations that come with MindSmarts.com. Now that MindSmarts.com is available, I plan to have them take the training. How is that for trust?

—Amin Bata
RE investor

I am the owner of Enhanced Wellness, LLC, in Jackson, Mississippi. As the owner of a wellness business, I have been a student of the brain for many years. Although Kep Kepner is not a brain scientist, he has teamed up with the Center for BrainHealth at the University of Texas at Dallas to apply their high-performance brain protocols to the business community. MindSmarts.com is armed with over 600 clinical studies from over 100 neuroscientists to back up the results from High-Performance Brain Training.

His information, when coupled with his business acumen, will help people reach the goals set out in their roadmap. Kep and his office are currently helping us with a substantial issue facing us, causing us to think deeply and broadly to come up with a solution. Since we have been working with Kep, our revenues have grown by about 50% and our gross profit by a similar amount.

—Kelly Engelmann
Enhanced Wellness

In the many years that KepnerCPA has been our CPA, our business has been through many substantial changes that coincided with family changes as well. Kep has always been able to clearly describe alternatives for the problems facing our business and the transition of responsibilities from me to my son. As any of us in business know, we must have someone who will give us the unvarnished truth and help us with an objective and independent view of our business.

The High-Performance Brain Training protocols are consistent with what business owners like me need to navigate the complex, ever-changing business world. He laughs and tells me about how I created enough inventory out of nothing for a new store location. Truth be told, he helped me do that.

—Mahmoud Kharrat
Kharrat Enterprises, Inc.

We own a thriving software business and a substantial direct mail shop in Dallas. KepnerCPA has been our CPA for many years and not only provides guidance on financial and tax matters but has applied his innovative knowledge and practices to our business. During the time we have worked with Kep, our business has grown 600%. When we encounter special circumstances, he is able to apply his protocols and technology to our business.

Although we have not yet learned his Brain Performance protocols, we are eager to embrace them and look forward to being front row and center when he presents his work at the Aspen Idea Festival. As we are learning about his High-Performance Brain Training, we can clearly see how it has been an active part of his consulting over the years. We highly recommend KepnerCPA and their MindSmarts Advisory services.

—Chele Butler, President
Barbara Morris, CEO
Fusemind, Inc.

While going through substantial changes in my life, the High-Performance Brain Training protocols helped me understand what was happening and helped me make effective decisions. Thanks, Kep.

—Evie Wise
Wise Insurance Group

As a financial advisor, my clients often identify "achieving a successful retirement" as their most important financial goal. Sometimes these clients own a business and want to retire. The business owner faces unique challenges in creating a retirement plan. Frequently, the value of the business and the owner's other assets are not adequate to create a viable retirement. This is where KepnerCPA comes in. Kep Kepner and his team at KepnerCPA advise business clients on how to increase the value of their business using his MindSmarts Advisory program.

Several years ago, Kep incorporated High-Performance Brain Training from the Center for BrainHealth at the University of Texas at Dallas into his business advisory program to accelerate results for his business clients. His MindSmarts Advisory program is now designed to help business owners leverage their own brain horsepower to make better business decisions. The MindSmarts program includes a client roadmap with structural components designed to grow a business from the inside out, not just adding sales. I became one of the first users and highly recommend it.

—James Lehman, CRPC®, AAMS®
Private Wealth Advisor

Made in the USA
Las Vegas, NV
14 May 2025